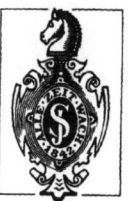

Martin Kaltenbach · Christian Vallbracht (Eds.)

Interventional Cardiology Frankfurt 1990

- **Rotational Angioplasty**
- **Coronary Balloon Angioplasty**
- **Coarctation of the Aorta**
- **Valvuloplasty**
- **Catheter Closure of Patent Ductus**
- **Appendix**

Springer-Verlag Berlin Heidelberg GmbH

Professor Dr. med. Martin Kaltenbach
Dr. med. Christian Vallbracht

Klinikum der
Johann Wolfgang Goethe-Universität Frankfurt
Zentrum der Inneren Medizin, Abteilung für Kardiologie
Theodor-Stern-Kai 7, D-6000 Frankfurt

ISBN 978-3-540-53156-2   ISBN 978-3-662-12117-7 (eBook)
DOI 10.1007/978-3-662-12117-7

2119/3145-543210

Contents

Introduction

Evolution of Angioplasty 2
M. KALTENBACH and C. VALLBRACHT

Rotational Angioplasty

Rotationsangioplastik –
Ein neues Katheterverfahren 8
M. KALTENBACH und C. VALLBRACHT

Rotationsangioplastik – Ein neues Verfahren
zur Gefäßwiedereröffnung und -erweiterung.
Experimentelle Befunde 11
C. VALLBRACHT, J. KRESS, M. SCHWEITZER,
M. SCHNEIDER, TH. WENDT, M. ZIEMEN, J. KOLLATH,
W. BAMBERG und M. KALTENBACH

Rotationsangioplastik – Erste klinische Ergebnisse
bei peripheren Gefäßverschlüssen 15
C. VALLBRACHT, M. SCHWEITZER, J. KRESS,
W. BAMBERG, J. KOLLATH, D. LIERMANN, C. PAASCH,
K. RAUBER, F. J. ROTH, J. PRIGNITZ, W. BEINBORN,
H. LANDGRAF, H. K. BREDDIN, W. SCHOOP,
und M. KALTENBACH

Rotationsangioplastik – Wiedereröffnung
chronischer Arterienverschlüsse mit einem
langsam rotierenden Katheter 21
C. VALLBRACHT, D. LIERMANN, I. PRIGNITZ, B. SÜSS,
H. AWISZUS, C. PAASCH, H. LANDGRAF, W. BEINBORN,
G. STICKELMANN, J. KOLLATH, F. J. ROTH, W. SCHOOP,
H. K. BREDDIN und M. KALTENBACH

Reopening of Chronic Coronary Artery Occlusions
by Low Speed Rotational Angioplasty 26
M. KALTENBACH and C. VALLBRACHT

Abstracts

Low Speed Rotational Angioplasty in Chronic
Coronary Artery Obstructions 35
M. KALTENBACH and C. VALLBRACHT

Medium-term Results After Reopening Chronic
Coronary Artery Obstructions by Low Speed
Rotational Angioplasty 36
M. KALTENBACH and C. VALLBRACHT

Low Speed Rotational Angioplasty in Chronic
Peripheral Occlusions – First Long-term Results ... 37
C. VALLBRACHT, F. J. ROTH, D. LIERMANN,
H. LANDGRAF, J. KOLLATH, W. SCHOOP,
and M. KALTENBACH

Coronary Balloon Angioplasty

Long Wire Technique – Experience
with 1000 Procedures 38
M. KALTENBACH, C. VALLBRACHT and G. KOBER

Koronarangioplastik – Ist das Rezidivrisiko
am Tage des Eingriffes voraussagbar?
Eine prospektive Untersuchung 42
C. VALLBRACHT, H. KLEPZIG jr., H. HOIN,
M. KALTENBACH und G. KOBER

Recognition of Restenosis: Can Patients be Defined
in Whom the Exercise-ECG Result Makes
Angiographic Restudy Unnecessary? 47
C. KADEL, T. STRECKER, M. KALTENBACH
and G. KOBER

Results of Repeat Angiography up to Eight Years
Following Percutaneous Transluminal Angioplasty
.... 51
G. KOBER, C. VALLBRACHT, C. KADEL
and M. KALTENBACH

Mehrfachrezidive nach Ballondilatation –
Dilatieren oder operieren? 55
C. VALLBRACHT, G. KOBER, B. KUNKEL, R. HOPF,
H. SIEVERT und M. KALTENBACH

Analysis of 100 Emergency Aortocoronary Bypass
Operations After Percutaneous Transluminal
Coronary Angioplasty: Which Patients are at Risk
for Large Infarctions? 60
H. KLEPZIG jr., G. KOBER, P. SATTER
and M. KALTENBACH

Coarctation of the Aorta

Transluminale Angioplastik der
Aortenisthmusstenose bei Jugendlichen
und Erwachsenen 68
H. SIEVERT, W.-D. BUSSMANN, W. PFOMMER,
J. REUHL und M. KALTENBACH

Aortenaneurysma nach Dilatation einer
Aortenisthmusstenose 71
H. SIEVERT, J. REUHL, R. SCHRÄDER,
M. KALTENBACH und W.-D. BUSSMANN

Valvuloplasty

Long-term Results of Percutaneous Pulmonary
Valvuloplasty in adults 76
H. SIEVERT, G. KOBER; W.-D. BUSSMANN,
J. REUHL, G. CIESLINSKI, P. SATTER
and M. KALTENBACH

Retrograde Mitral Valvuloplasty –
A Further Approach to Ballon
Commissurotomy 81
H. SIEVERT, P. KRÄMER, M. KALTENBACH
and G. KOBER

Transluminale Valvuloplastik der nicht verkalkten
Aortenstenose: Akut- und Langzeitergebnisse 84
H. SIEVERT, P. KRÄMER, W.-D. BUSSMANN,
M. KALTENBACH und G. KOBER

Restenosis is a Common Feature of the
Angiographic Follow-up After Ballon Valvoplasty
of Calcified Aortic Stenoses 87
H. SIEVERT, P. KRÄMER, G. KOBER,
W.-D. BUSSMANN and M. KALTENBACH

Catheter Closure of Patent Ducuts

Ein Katheter zur Darstellung des Ductus arteriosus
persistens 92
H. SIEVERT, E. NIEMÖLLER, W.-D. BUSSMANN
G. KOBER, M. KALTENBACH mit techn. Ass. von
K. P. KÖHLER und W. BAMBERG

Visualization of the Patent Ductus by Means of
a New Low Pressure Ballon Catheter 95
H. SIEVERT, E. NIEMÖLLER, W.-D. BUSSMANN,
G. KOBER and M. KALTENBACH

Transfemoraler Ductus-Botalli-Verschluß 99
Akut- und Langzeitergebnisse
H. SIEVERT, E. NIEMÖLLER, K. P. KÖHLER,
W. BAMBERG, H. HANKE, P. SATTER, M. KALTENBACH
und W.-D. BUSSMANN

Appendix

Koronarschemata 106
(Coronary diagrams)

Introduction

Evolution of Angioplasty

M. KALTENBACH and C. VALLBRACHT

Angioplasty evolved through a series of very unusual ideas and their application to patients with atherosclerotic heart disease.

Charles Dotter and Melvin Judkins described in 1964 how peripheral arteries with atherosclerotic obstructions could be recanalized using catheters with increasing diameters fed over a wire. They demonstrated that the reopened vessels were not necessarily reoccluded by thrombus formation and stayed open in the majority of patients (Fig. 1).

had become feasible only after Mason Sones had pioneered selective coronary arteriography in 1957 and René Favoloro aortocoronary bypass surgery in 1967.

John Simpson introduced 1982 the steerable balloon catheter. In 1984 the steerable system was expanded to the long-wire technique. With this technique coronary stenoses are passed by a free wire which is not hindered in any way by the balloon catheter, thus allowing optimal opacification and sensitive maneuvering during the process of passing coronary obstructions (Kaltenbach).

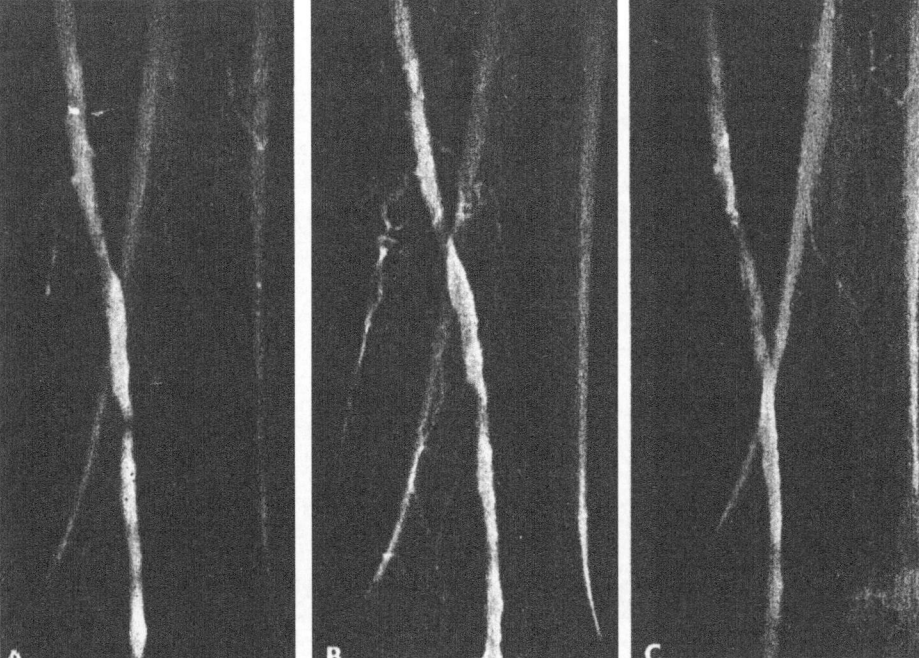

Fig. 1. Case 1 of the first published report of transluminal catheter dilatation by Charles T. Dotter and Melvin P. Judkins [1] in 1964

In 1973 Werner Porstmann introduced a nondistensible "corset" balloon. This instrument offered the possibility to widen an artery far beyond the diameter of the introduced catheter.

Andreas Grüntzig developed in 1974 the noncompliant balloon with a cylindrical shape of defined diameter resistant to high pressures. He demonstrated by systematic studies that the acute and long-term results achieved with this instrument in peripheral artery disease are beneficial. The first coronary angioplasty procedure was performed on September 16, 1977, in Zurich and a total of 6 patients were treated in 1977 in Zurich and Frankfurt (Fig. 2). This application of angioplasty to coronary artery disease

All the technical advances, achieved over 10 years have led to a 90 % success rate of coronary balloon angioplasty and a total of probably more than 300 000 procedures were performed in 1989. Clinical experience suggests that coronary angioplasty will become a still increasingly important technique for coronary revascularization in the 1990s and that the number of patients so treated is most likely to exceed the total revascularized by surgery. In the early years of coronary angioplasty it was estimated that 5 % of patients were treated by this procedure instead of undergoing surgery; today this figure has risen to between 30 and 50 %.

Coronary angioplasty 1977

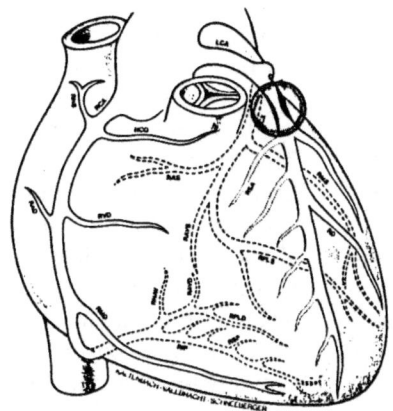

1 B. A., ♂, LAD, 9/16/1977, Zürich

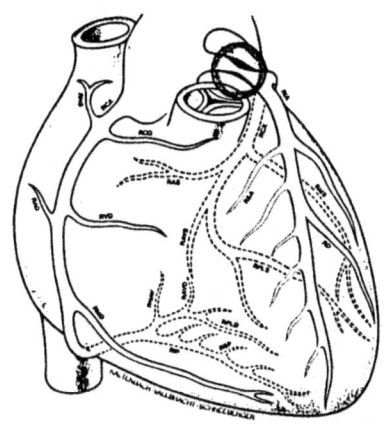

4 B. H., ♂, LM, 11/24/1977, Frankfurt

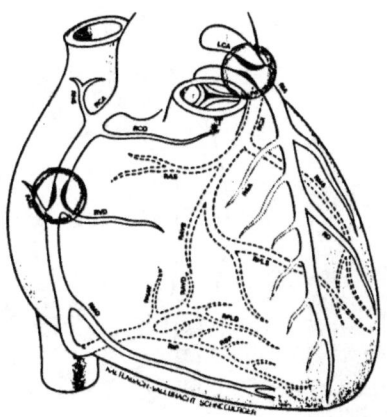

2 M. F., ♂, LM/RCA, 10/18/1977, Frankfurt

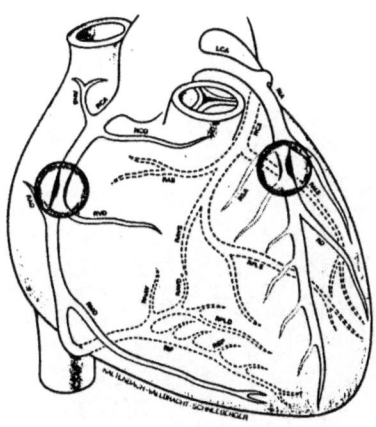

5 B. P., ♂, LAD, 12/13/1977, Zürich

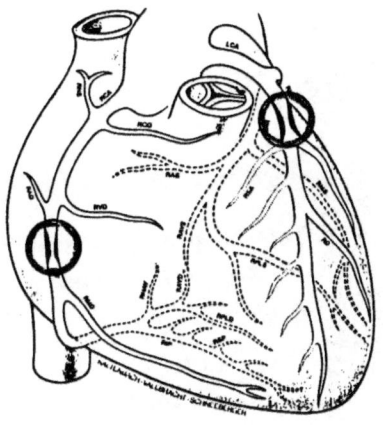

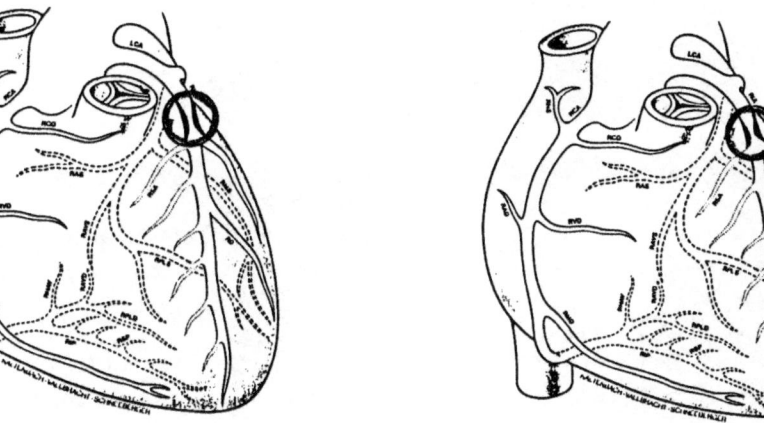

Fig. 2. Diagrams of the obstructions in the six patients who had angioplasty in 1977: two with single-vessel disease (*1, 6*), two with double-vessel disease (*3, 5*), and two with left main disease (*2, 4*)

3 B. A., ♂, LAD/RCA, 11/21/1977, Zürich

6 F. H., ♂, LAD, 12/20/1977, Zürich

This increase in the percentage of patients being treated with angioplasty is the consequence of improved techniques – better guide wires, better balloon catheters – and greater experience. More importantly, it is also the result of many observations over up to 10 years which show unequivocally that long-term prognosis is excellent if coronary artery stenosis does not recur within a few months after successful dilatation.

The atherosclerotic tissue is replaced by scar tissue which halts the progression of the disease. Late recurrences at the site of a previous angioplasty are rare, occurring in less than 1% of cases.

These findings constitute the most important lesson from our 10 years of experience with balloon angioplasty. They mean that long-term results are as good as those of *arterial* aortocoronary bypass surgery and are superior to those of venous bypass graft operations, which suffer from a reocclusion rate of about 50% at 10 years.

Thus, whenever there is reason to believe that angioplasty can be performed with a good chance of success (> 80%) and with low risk to the patient (< 1%), this procedure is to be preferred to surgery.

The challenges of the 1990s are two problems, namely restenosis and chronic occlusions.

Restenosis rate is still around 30%. Mechanical tools including the implantation of stents and medications for the prevention of restenosis have failed to reduce this rate substantially.

Experience with atherectomy performed with John Simpson's Atherocut catheter has confirmed the feasibility of this procedure in the coronary circulation, but restenosis rate is apparently not substantially reduced. In excentric stenoses, however, the results of atherectomy may be superior to those achieved with balloon angioplasty.

Chronic occlusions can only be reopened with presently available techniques in about 50%. The success rate markedly decreases in occlusions older than 6 months. This prevents the adequate treatment of patients who have continuing ischemia in the myocardium distal to a coronary occlusion. But also if coronary occlusion brings about the loss of collateral flow into myocardium supplied by other stenosed coronary arteries, the risk of angioplasty in these stenosed arteries is greatly increased. In such a situation coronary angioplasty of a critical stenosis can only be performed with low risk if the occlusion has been reopened. Even if chronically occluded coronary arteries are perfusing infarcted parts of the myocardium, reopening of such arteries might be of benefit. The re-

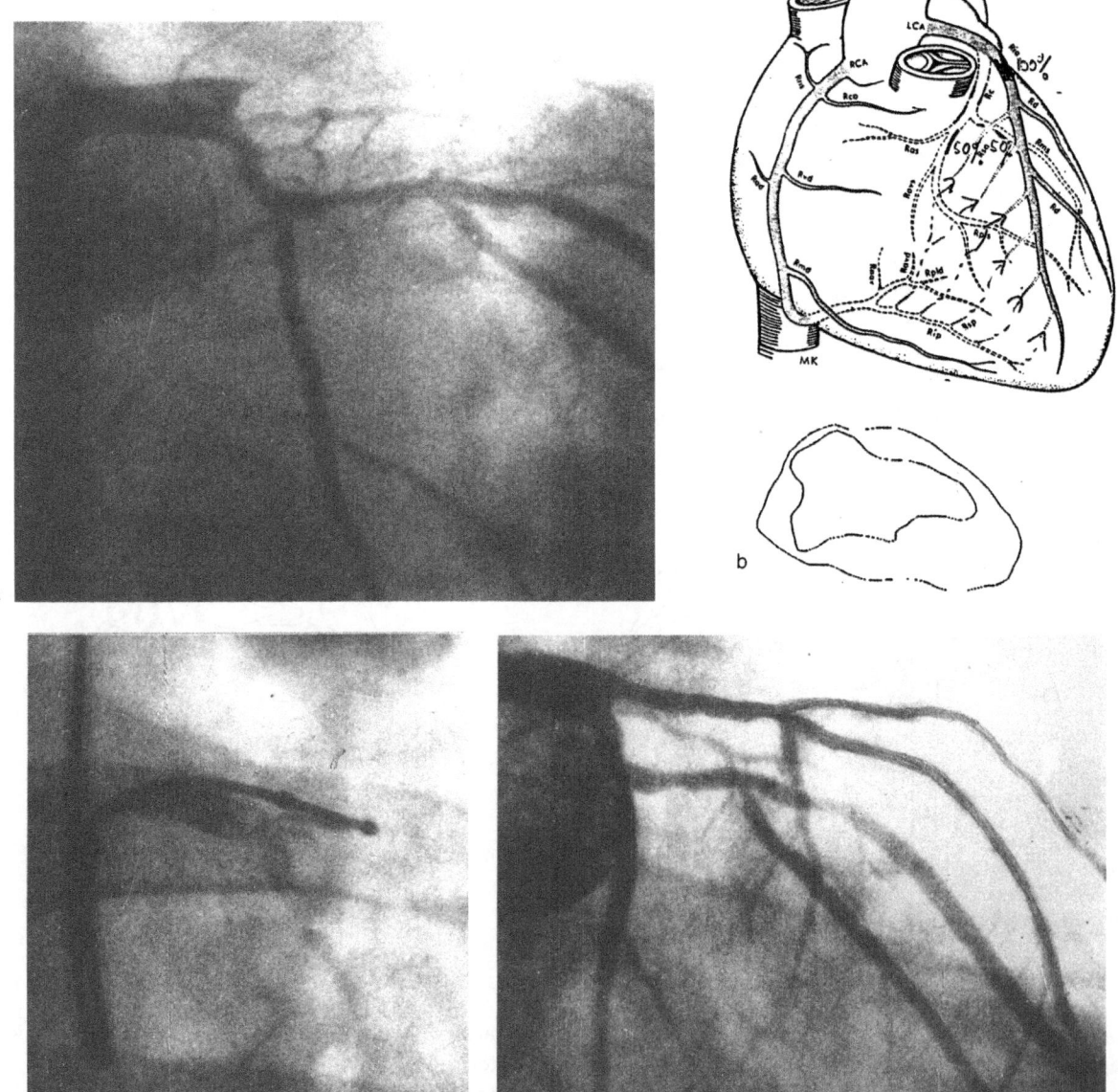

Fig. 3. a Chronic proximal occlusion of the LAD in a patient with stable angina pectoris. **b** Other vessels free, retrograde filling of the LAD from the RCA. Left ventricle shows only slight anterior hypokinesia. **c** Rotational catheter in the obstruction, contrast injection through the rotational catheter. **d** Recanalized LAD

Landmarks in the Development of Angioplasty

1964 Transluminal treatment of stenoses and short arterial occlusions using a new catheter system.
C. R. Dotter and M. P. Judkins [1] (Fig. 1)

1973 "Corset" balloon catheter for transluminal dilatation of iliac stenoses.
W. Porstmann [2]

1974 Nondistensible double-lumen balloon catheter for transluminal angioplasty of peripheral arterial stenoses.
A. Grüntzig [3]

1977 First coronary angioplasty in Zurich.
A. Grüntzig [4] (Fig. 2)

1977 First coronary angioplasty in Frankfurt.
M. Kaltenbach and G. Kober [4] (Fig. 2)

1982 The steerable technique for coronary angioplasty.
J. B. Simpson [5]

1984 The long-wire technique for coronary angioplasty
M. Kaltenbach [6]

1985 Transluminal atherectomy.
J. B. Simpson [7]

1986 The monorail technique for coronary angioplasty.
T. Bonzel [8]

1987 Low-speed rotational angioplasty.
M. Kaltenbach and C. Vallbracht [9] (Fig. 3)

maining myocardium may become better and collaterals arising from these arteries can become important, if coronary artery disease progresses in other branches.

Reopening of chronic occlusions can be performed with conventional guide wires. Thick guide wires are applied, wires can be stiffened by the use of recanalization catheters. If a guide wire can be advanced through the occlusion, a variety of "over the wire" techniques can be applied. Beside balloon angioplasty, hot-tip catheters, high-speed drilling instruments (as described by Auth and Ritchie), and laser catheters are used. Application of such techniques in chronic occlusions which can*not* be penetrated by a wire remains, however, problematical (Kensey 1986), particularly in tortuous vessels which can easily be perforated.

If the occlusion cannot be crossed with a guide wire, a new technique is low-speed rotational angioplasty (Kaltenbach and Vallbracht 1987). Passage of the occlusion is performed in an atraumatic fashion, and the technique has no tendency to perforate the vessel wall. It is performed with a blunt and soft catheter. The stainless steel catheter is designed in such a way that extreme flexibility is combined with high torque control. The catheter is rotated at a low speed of about 200 rpm. This speed is sufficient to abolish friction. Therefore sensitive movements in the longitudinal direction can be performed. During passage of the obstruction contrast injection can be made through the rotating catheter.

Applicability of rotational angioplasty has been demonstrated in > 150 patients with chronic peripheral occlusions. Occlusions existing for more than one year and extending over a length of more than 30 cm can be reopened successfully in 80% of cases. No vessel wall perforations have occurred.

After technical refining and miniaturization, the technique is applied to chronic coronary artery obstructions. Many chronic occlusions not responding to conventional techniques can be reopened with low-speed rotational angioplasty. Experience in more than 70 patients shows the applicability to chronic occlusions exceeding 6 months. The new technique will allow us to expand nonsurgical revascularization to a group of patients who so far have been candidates only for surgery (Fig. 3).

References

1. Dotter CT, Judkins MP (1964) Transluminal treatment of arteriosclerotic obstruction: description of a new technique and a preliminary report of its application. Circulation 30: 654
2. Porstmann W (1973) Ein neuer Korsett-Ballonkatheter zur transluminalen Rekanalisation nach Dotter unter besonderer Berücksichtigung von Obliterationen an den Beckenarterien. Radiol Diagn 14: 239
3. Grüntzig A, Hopf H (1974) Perkutane Rekanalisation chronischer arterieller Verschlüsse mit einem neuen Dilatationskatheter. Modifikation der Dotter-Technik. Dtsch Med Wochenschr 99: 2502
4. Grüntzig A (1978) Transluminal dilatation of coronary artery stenoses (letter) Lancet I: 263
5. Simpson JB, Blaim DS, Robert E, Harrison DC (1982) A new catheter system for coronary angioplasty. Am J Cardiol 49: 1216
6. Kaltenbach M (1984) Neue Technik zur Ballondilatation von Kranzgefäßverengungen. Z Kardiol 73: 669
7. Simpson JB, Johnson DE, Thapliyal HV, Marks DS, Braden LJ (1985) Transluminal atherectomy. A new approach to the treatment of atherosclerotic vascular disease. Circulation 72 (Suppl II) 111–146
8. Bonzel T, Wollschläger H, Just H (1986) Ein neues Kathetersystem zur mechanischen Dilatation von Koronarstenosen mit austauschbaren intrakoronaren Kathetern, höherem Kontrastmittelfluß und verbesserter Steuerbarkeit. Biomed Technik 21: 195
9. Kaltenbach M, Vallbracht C (1987) Rotationsangioplastik – ein neues Katheterverfahren. Fortschr Med 105: 412

Rotational Angioplasty

Rotationsangioplastik – Ein neues Katheterverfahren

Rekanalisation bei bislang nur operativ behandelbaren Patienten in Aussicht

M. KALTENBACH und C. VALLBRACHT

Die von Grüntzig begründete Angioplastik mit Hilfe von Ballonkathetern [1] hat die Durchführung nichtoperativer Revaskularisationsmaßnahmen in einem noch vor wenigen Jahren für undenkbar gehaltenen Umfang ermöglicht. Das Verfahren hat sich besonders bei koronaren Durchblutungsstörungen im Lauf von zehn Jahren rapid verbreitet. Diese Verbreitung ist hauptsächlich deswegen gerechtfertigt, weil die jetzt beurteilbaren Langzeitergebnisse größtenteils ausgezeichnet sind.

Die Anwendung der Ballondilatation findet derzeit ihre Begrenzung bei Gefäßverschlüssen und extrem engen oder weit distal in stark gekrümmten Gefäßabschnitten lokalisierten Stenosen, die mit dem Ballonkatheter nicht passiert werden können. Ein neues mechanisches Verfahren erscheint für die Anwendung in solchen Situationen erfolgversprechend. Die im folgenden zu beschreibenden experimentellen Befunde und erste klinische Erfahrungen lassen erwarten, daß damit die Anwendung der Angioplastik in Zukunft möglicherweise noch wesentlich erweitert werden kann.

Zusammenfassung

Es wird ein neues Kathetersystem beschrieben, das aus einem rotationsstabilen und zugleich sehr flexiblen Katheter sowie einem stufenlos regelbaren Antrieb besteht. Experimentelle und erste klinische Erfahrungen lassen erwarten, daß das neue System Eigenschaften besitzt, die möglicherweise nichtoperative Revaskularisationsmaßnahmen auch bei Patienten erlauben, die bisher nur operativ behandelt werden können.

Summary: Rotatory Angioplasty – A New Catheter Procedure for Non-operative Revascularization

A new catheter system is described, which consists of a rotatory-stable and at the same time very flexible catheter with an adjustable power supply. Experimental and the first clinical experience show that the new system has qualities, which will probably enable non-operative revascularization in patients, who could otherwise only be treated operatively.

Schlüsselwörter: Koronarangioplastik – Katheterdilatation – neue Technik
Keywords: Coronary angioplasty – catheter dilation – new technique

Methode

Neuentwickelter Katheter

Der Rotationskatheter besteht aus einer mehrgängigen Schraubenfeder. Diese ist aus hochwertigem V2A-Stahl von 0,1 bis 0,3 mm Durchmesser hergestellt (Abb. 1). Es werden zwei bis acht, in der Regel vier Schraubengänge gewickelt. Der Drahtdurchmesser ist den Katheterdurchmessern angepaßt. Diese liegen in der Regel zwischen 1 und 3 mm.

Die Oberfläche des Katheters ist mit einer Polyolefin-Schrumpfschlauchschicht hoher Elastizität oder mit einer aufgespritzten Teflonschicht überzogen. Das distale Katheterende weist einen stumpfen Kopf auf oder besteht aus einem elastischen, in seinem Durchmesser veränderbaren Glied. Der stumpfe Kopf dient zur Wiedereröffnung von Gefäßverschlüssen, das erweiterbare Endglied zur rotierenden Gefäßerweiterung.

Der proximale Katheterteil wird mit einem Draht oder einem Luer-System verschlossen. Die Abdichtung zum Führungskatheter erfolgt mit einer Kupplung, die eine freie Rotierbarkeit gewährleistet. Eine zweite Kupplung gestattet die Übertragung von Längsbewegungen auf den Katheter während elektromotorischer Rotation (Abb. 2, 3).

Der Katheter besitzt infolge seiner extrem dünnen Wand ein weites Lumen, durch das Führungsdrähte bzw. Wechseldrähte eingeführt werden können. Er kann auch doppellumig ausgeführt werden, so daß nur der innere Teil rotiert. Die Rotation erfolgt über einen Elektromotor, dessen Drehzahl stufenlos regelbar ist. Er ist mit einem Vor- und Rücklaufschalter sowie einer Überlastungskupplung ausgestattet. Es besteht zusätzlich die Möglichkeit, motorisch axiale Bewegungen zu erzeugen.

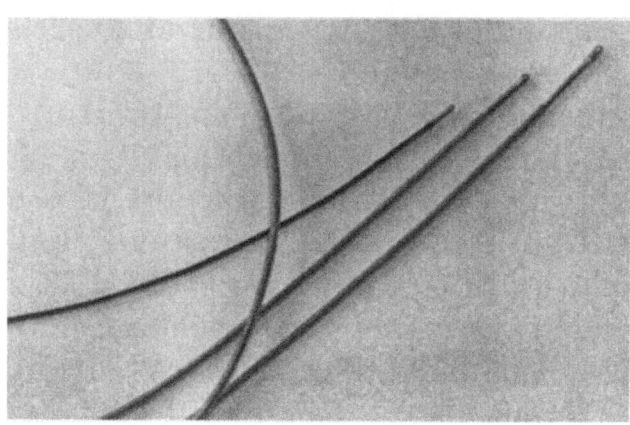

Abb. 1. Rotationskatheter verschiedener Durchmesser

Sonderdruck aus Fortschr der Medizin, 21: 412–414, 1987, Urban & Vogel München

Der Rotationskatheter wird durch einen üblichen Führungskatheter eingeführt. Er kann allein verwendet werden oder einen nicht rotierenden Mantel tragen, der aus Kunststoff besteht oder wiederum aus einer mehrgängigen Schraubenfeder von besonders geringer Wanddicke.

Ergebnisse

Im Experiment keine Wandschädigung

In postmortalen stenosierten Arterien verursachte die Einführung und Applikation des Rotationskathetersystems keine erkennbaren Wandschädigungen oder Dissektionen. Chronisch verschlossene Arterien konnten auch im Bereich langstreckiger und stark verkalkter Verschlüsse wiedereröffnet werden. Wandperforationen durch den Rotationskatheter traten nicht auf.

Der neugeschaffene Kanal zeigte angiographisch, angioskopisch und histologisch relativ glatte Begrenzungen. Die Erweiterung des neugeschaffenen Kanals erfolgte durch Ballondilatation.

Wiedereröffnung chronischer Verschlüsse

Vorläufige Ergebnisse bei Patienten mit arteriellen Durchblutungsstörungen der Beine zeigten die Möglichkeit der Wiedereröffnung chronischer Verschlüsse, auch wenn diese bei vorausgegangenen Eingriffen mit konventioneller Technik unmöglich war bzw. zur Gefäßwanddissektion geführt hatte.

Diskussion

Erstmals langsame Rotation eingesetzt

Die Angioplastik mit langsam rotierenden Kathetersystemen wurde bislang nicht beschrieben. Sie unterscheidet sich von anderen Rotationskathetersystemen sowohl technisch als auch in bezug auf die Zielrichtung und die zugrundeliegenden pathophysiologischen Vorgänge. Das Grundgerüst des von uns verwendeten Katheters aus einer mehrgängigen Stahl-Schraubenfeder verbindet eine hohe Drehfestigkeit mit dünner Wand und extremer Flexibilität. Es gestattet, Längsbewegungen ohne Stau-

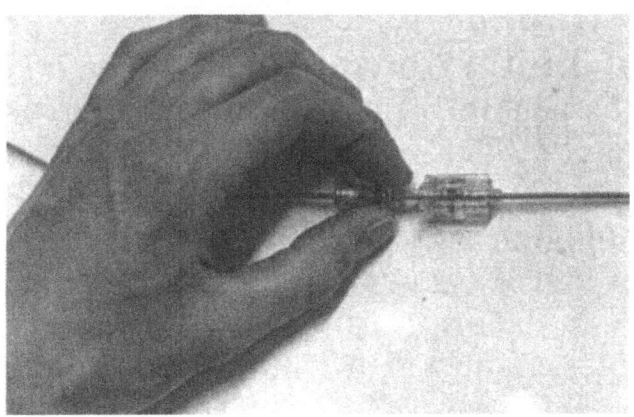

Abb. 2. Rotationskupplung für die Übertragung von Längsbewegungen

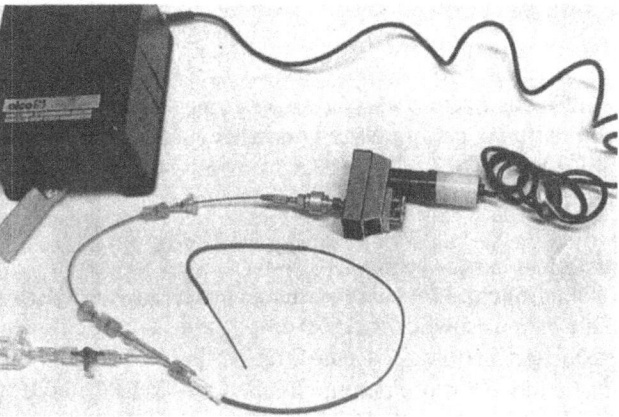

Abb. 3. Rotationskatheter mit stufenlos regelbarem Antrieb. Spannfutter mit Rutschkupplung, Rotationskupplungen und Anschlußstück. Der Führungskatheter wurde zur besseren Sichtbarmachung des Rotationskatheters im mittleren Areal entfernt

chungsverlust und weitgehend reibungsfrei zu übertragen. Die Rotationsgeschwindigkeit liegt um 100 bis 1000 U/min, im Gegensatz zu »Bohrkathetern« mit 50 000 bis 150 000 U/min [2, 5].

Zur Wiedereröffnung chronischer Gefäßverschlüsse erwies sich ein parabolisch abgerundeter stumpfer Katheterkopf als gut geeignet. Dieser erlaubt eine weitgehend atraumatische Gefäßwiedereröffnung, die mit einer stumpfen Präparation vergleichbar ist und – im Gegensatz zu Systemen beispielsweise mit der Anwendung von Laserstrahlen – keine Tendenz zur Wandperforation aufweist. Der Katheter findet seinen Weg durch die Gewebepartien plastisch-weicher Konsistenz, während die elastische Gefäßwand nicht penetriert werden kann.

Verdrängung und Kompression statt Abrasion

Der pathophysiologische Ansatz ist dadurch von Rotationskathetersystemen mit hoher Drehzahl, bei denen das distale Katheterende einen Bohrkopf trägt, der mit Düsen bzw. kleinen Diamanten bestückt ist, um einen Bohr- bzw. Fräsvorgang mit Abrasion arteriosklerotischen Materials zu bewirken, grundlegend unterschieden. Als pathophysiologischer Grundvorgang wird die Verschlußwiedereröffnung und Gefäßweitung durch Verdrängung und Kompression arteriosklerotischen Materials angesehen. Wie in früheren Untersuchungen an postmortalem atherosklerotischen Gewebe nachgewiesen, läßt sich eine plastische Verformung und Volumenverkleinerung von Atheromen durch Flüssigkeitsabpressung bzw. -verlagerung erzielen [4]. Dementsprechend handelt es sich bei unserer Methode um einen Kompressions- und Verdrängungsvorgang. Die langsame Drehzahl des stumpfen Kopfes verleiht dem Katheter die Fähigkeit, dem Verlauf des ursprünglichen Gefäßkanals zu folgen. Der rotierende Kopf von relativ großem Außendurchmesser dringt in die weichsten, plastischen Gewebeanteile ein, während elastische Elemente, wie die Gefäßwand, ihm ausweichen. Die axiale Reibung wird durch die elektromotorische Rotation weitgehend aufgehoben, so daß Längsbewegungen feinfühlig übertragbar sind.

Mehr Verschlüsse erreichbar

Vorläufige klinische Ergebnisse an Patienten mit peripherer arterieller Verschlußkrankheit bestätigen die günstigen Eigenschaften des neuen Kathetersystems. Eine Wiedereröffnung gelingt unter Umständen auch beim Vorliegen atheromatöser arterieller Verschlüsse, die mit konventionellen Verfahren nicht wiedereröffnet werden konnten. Wandpenetrationen oder -perforationen wurden nicht beobachtet.

In experimentellen Untersuchungen wies der entstandene neue Kanal sowohl makroskopisch wie auch angioskopisch und histologisch eine ungewöhnlich glatte Oberfläche auf. Er war einer anschließenden Weiterdilatation durch konventionelle Ballonkatheter unter Verwendung der Langdrahttechnik [3] gut zugänglich.

Hoffnung auf Indikationserweiterung

Falls sich die bisherigen Erfahrungen an einem größeren Krankengut bestätigen, wird die neue Kathetertechnologie die Indikation zur Angioplastik erheblich erweitern können. Das gilt möglicherweise auch für Kranzarterienverschlüsse, die z. Zt. nicht mit ausreichender Erfolgsaussicht angegangen werden können. Die Erfolgsrate ist selbst bei Verschlüssen von weniger als drei Monaten Dauer niedrig und beträgt nur etwa 50%. Auch manche hochgradigen Stenosen sind mit bisheriger Technik nicht erweiterbar, weil sie sich mit dem Ballonkatheter nicht passieren lassen. In einigen Fällen gelingt die Passage überhaupt nicht, in anderen kann zwar der Führungsdraht, jedoch nicht der Ballonkatheter durch die Stenose vorgeschoben werden. Das ist besonders bei stark gewundenem Gefäßverlauf, z. B. in der distalen rechten Kranzarterie oder im Circumflexa-Bereich der Fall. Auch in dieser Situation ist die neue Technik erfolgversprechend. Eine andere Begrenzung der Indikation liegt derzeit vor, wenn ein Gefäß stenosiert, ein anderes dagegen verschlossen ist. Auch wenn das verschlossene Gefäß nicht eröffnet werden muß, weil es zu einem Infarktareal führt, ist der Eingriff bei solchen Kranken nur mit deutlich erhöhtem Risiko durchführbar; ein durch den Dilatationsvorgang entstehender plötzlicher Gefäßverschluß in dem stenosierten Gefäß kann nicht kompensiert werden, weil das kollateralengebende Gefäß verschlossen ist.

Wenn mit der neuen Technik in solchen Fällen zuerst das verschlossene Gefäß wiedereröffnet werden kann, ist der Eingriff mit geringerem Risiko durchführbar und eine vollständige Revaskularisation zu erreichen.

Das beschriebene neue Kathetersystem bietet insgesamt Ansätze, um in Zukunft möglicherweise nichtoperative Revaskularisationsmaßnahmen auch bei Patienten durchführen zu können, die bisher nur operativ behandelbar waren.

Literatur

1. Grüntzig A: Transluminal dilatation of coronary artery stenosis. Lancet 1978/I: 263
2. Hansen DD, Auth DC, Vracko R, Ritchie JL: In vivo mechanical thrombolysis in subacute canine arterial occlusion. Circulation 72, Suppl, abstr. III-469, 1875 (1985)
3. Kaltenbach M: The long wire technique – a new technique for steerable balloon catheter dilatation of coronary artery stenoses. Eur Heart J 5, 1004–1009 (1984)
4. Kaltenbach M, Beyer J, Walter S, Klepzig H, Schmidts L: Prolonged application of pressure in transluminal coronary angioplasty. Cath Cardiovasc Diagn 10, 213–219 (1984)
5. Kensey K, Nash J, Abrahams C, Lake K, Zarins CK: Circulation 74, Suppl, abstr. II-457, 1821 (1986)

Für die Verfasser:
Prof. Dr. med. M. Kaltenbach, Zentrum der Inneren Medizin, Abteilung für Kardiologie, Klinikum der Universität, Theodor-Stern-Kai 7, D-6000 Frankfurt am Main

Rotationsangioplastik – Ein neues Verfahren zur Gefäßwiedereröffnung und -erweiterung. Experimentelle Befunde

C. Vallbracht, J. Kress, M. Schweitzer, M. Schneider, Th. Wendt, M. Ziemen, J. Kollath, W. Bamberg und M. Kaltenbach

Low speed rotational angioplasty – a new technique to reopen and dilate chronic vessel occlusions. Experimental results.

Summary: 16 fresh postmortem specimens of human femoral and popliteal arteries with severe atherosclerosis were removed and angiography was performed. Eight vessels were completely occluded and eight showed stenoses of up to 60 %. All occluded vessels were heavily calcified. The duration of occlusion, estimated according to the patient's history, ranged from 1 to 2 years. In one case, a duration of 18 months was documented by angiography. The lengths of the occlusions were between 5 and 12 cm. A rotating catheter was introduced through a 9F guiding catheter. All stenosed vessels were passed and seven out of eight occluded vessels, in which passage was not possible using conventional wires, were successfully reopened at low speed rotation of 200 rpm. Angiography, as well as histology, showed no perforation, and angioscopy revealed a smooth surface of the new channel. In three vessels this new channel was dilated with a balloon catheter and in one with an elastic element under rotation. It is concluded that with the new technique it is possible to reopen totally occluded human arteries which cannot be passed by conventional methods.

Zusammenfassung: 16 Leichenarterien (A. femoralis sup. und A. poplitea) mit schwerer Arteriosklerose wurden präpariert und angiographisch dargestellt. 8 Arterien waren komplett verschlossen und zeigten deutliche Verkalkungen, 8 Arterien zeigten Lumeneinengungen bis 60 %. Das Verschlußalter konnte auf 12–24 Monate geschätzt, in einem Fall mit mindestens 18 Monaten angiographisch dokumentiert werden. Die Verschlußlängen lagen zwischen 4 und 12 cm. Über einen 9F-Führungskatheter wurde eine biegsame, mit Polyolefin überschrumpfte Welle aus 4 × 0,2 mm-V2A-Schraubendrähten eingeführt. Angetrieben von einem Elektromotor wurden die stenosierten Arterien passiert. 7 von 8 verschlossenen Arterien, die mit herkömmlichen Führungsdrähten nicht zu eröffnen waren, wurden erfolgreich wiedereröffnet. Perforationen traten in keinem Fall auf. Die angiographische, histologische und angioskopische Kontrolle dokumentierte einen relativ glatten neuen Kanal, der bei 3 Arterien mit einem herkömmlichen Ballonkatheter und bei 2 Arterien mit einem rotierenden elastischen Drahtelement geweitet wurde. Es wird gefolgert, daß mit der neuen Technik arterielle

Verschlüsse passiert werden können, die mit herkömmlichen Methoden nicht zu eröffnen sind.

Einleitung

Die nichtoperative Erweiterung arteriosklerotisch verengter Blutgefäße, von Charles Dotter 1964 erstmals an peripheren Arterien durchgeführt [2] und von Andreas Grüntzig durch Entwicklung der Ballondilatation entscheidend weiterentwickelt [5], gehört heute zur klinischen Routine vieler Zentren in der ganzen Welt. Neben den Arterien der unteren Extremität [5, 13] spielen besonders Koronarstenosen [4], Stenosen der Nierenarterien [1] und zunehmend auch Gehirnarterien [10] eine wichtige Rolle. Gleichzeitig wurde das Prinzip der Dehnung einer Einengung mit Hilfe eines Ballonkatheters auf andere Hohlsysteme wie den Ösophagus oder abführende Harnwege übertragen, und weitere Anwendungsgebiete sind denkbar (z. B. Prostatahypertrohpie).

Durch wesentliche technische Weiterentwicklungen wie die Einführung steuerbarer Ballonkatheter [12] können heute ca. 90 % aller angegangenen Arterienverengungen erfolgreich erweitert werden [1, 9].

Die Grenzen liegen bei hochgradigen, mit dem Führungsdraht oder Ballonkatheter nicht zu passierenden Stenosen und besonders bei Gefäßverschlüssen. Periphere Gefäß-

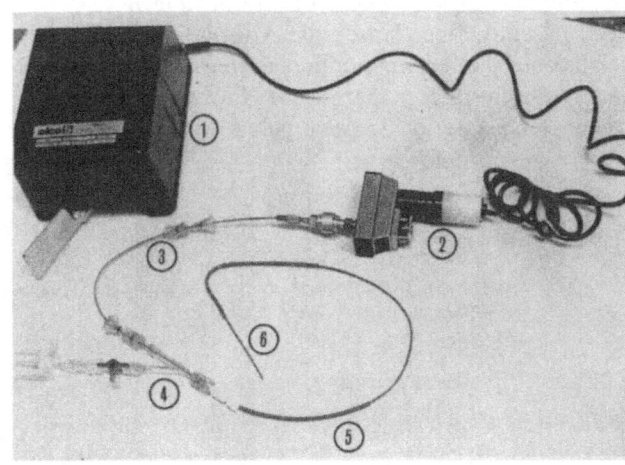

Abb. 1. Rotationsangioplastik. **1.** Impulsgeber, **2.** Elektromotor, **3.** Rotationsadapter, **4.** Rotationsschleuse, **5.** Führungskatheter, **6.** Rotationswelle

Schlüsselwörter: transluminale Angioplastik, periphere Gefäßverschlüsse

Sonderdruck aus Z Kardiologie, 76: 608–611, 1987, Springer Berlin Heidelberg

verschlüsse über 10 cm Länge und subakute Koronarverschlüsse sind bisher nur in etwa 50 % der Fälle erweiterbar [9, 13], wobei mit zunehmender Verschlußdauer und nachweisbaren Verkalkungen die Chance einer Wiedereröffnung sinkt.

Von Kaltenbach wurde 1985 eine neue Technik beschrieben, bei der eine rotierende Welle benutzt wird [6]. Diese gestattet mit einem stumpfen Kopf die schonende Wiedereröffnung eines Verschlusses. Der entstehende Kanal kann entweder mit herkömmlichen Ballonkathetern oder mit einem speziellen elastischen Element rotierend geweitet werden.

Technik

Eine biegsame Welle von 1,4 mm Außendurchmesser, bestehend aus vier Schraubendrähten aus 0,2-mm-V2A-Stahl, mit einem Innenlumen zur Einführung eines Wechseldrahtes und abgerundeter stumpfer Spitze, wird von einem Elektromotor angetrieben. Die Außenwand der Welle ist entweder mit einem Polyolefin-Schrumpfschlauch hoher Elastizität oder einer Teflonschicht überzogen. Der Elektromotor ist stufenlos von 0 bis 1200 U/min regelbar, mit Links- und Rechtslauf sowie einer Rutschkupplung ausgestattet. Die Drehgeschwindigkeit wird über den Fußschalter des Trafos geregelt.

Zur klinischen Anwendung wurde eine spezielle Rotationsschleuse entwickelt, die die freie Drehung der Welle bei dichtem Abschluß des Blutgefäßes gestattet, gleichzeitig Longitudinalbewegungen und die Perfusion des Führungskatheters mit 2000 E Heparin/h und 100 000 E Urokinase/h erlaubt. Zur manuellen Führung der Welle dient ein Rotationsadapter, der die longitudinalen Bewegungen der Welle bei ungehinderter Rotation erlaubt. Alle Teile mit Ausnahme des Trafos sind gassterilisierbar (Abb. 1).

Methodik der experimentellen Untersuchungen
Bei 16 Obduktionen wurde die Arteria femoralis superficialis oder die Arteria poplitea entfernt, bei denen sich anamnestische oder palpatorische Hinweise auf eine fortgeschrittene Arteriosklerose ergaben.

Die Gefäße wurden weitgehend frei präpariert und größere Seitenäste unterbunden. Mit Hilfe eines 9-French-Führungskatheters wurde das Gefäß zunächst angiographisch dargestellt und der Befund auf Cinefilm (Filmgeschwindigkeit 25 Bilder/s) dokumentiert.

Nach erfolgter Rotationsangioplastik wurde erneut angiographisch kontrolliert. Bei 4 Arterien wurde daraufhin die histologische Aufarbeitung mit Serienschnitten im Abstand von 5 mm vorgenommen. Bei 2 Gefäßen wurden zusätzlich der Verschluß sowie der neu entstandene Kanal mit Hilfe eines 1,5-mm-Angioskops (Edwards-Laboratories) sichtbar gemacht und auf Videofilm dokumentiert.

Ergebnisse

Acht Arterien zeigten in der angiographischen Darstellung komplette Verschlüsse des Lumens; alle 8 wiesen erhebliche Verkalkungen auf. Nach anamnestischen Angaben konnte das Alter der Verschüsse auf 12–14 Monate festgelegt werden; in einem Fall war die Verschlußdauer von mindestens 18 Monaten angiograpisch zu belegen (Voruntersuchung). Die Länge der Verschlüsse lag zwischen 4 und 12 cm. Die übrigen 8 Gefäße zeigten Lumeneinengungen bis 60% linearer Durchmesserminderung.

Über den 9-French-Führungskatheter wurde die Rotationswelle eingeführt. Unter langsamer Drehung bis maximal 200 U/min und manuellem Vor- und Zurückführen mittels des Rotationsadapters wurden die 8 stenosierten Gefäße passiert. Dissektionen oder Perforationen traten nicht auf.

Sieben von acht komplett verschlossenen Gefäßen konnten erfolgreich wiedereröffnet werden; bei einem Gefäß war ein völlig verkalktes Endstück von 0,5 cm Länge nicht zu passieren.

Die angiographische Kontrolle zeigte auch hier keine Perforationen; bei einem Gefäß war eine Dissektion zu erkennen, die erfolgreich umgangen werden konnte.

Der durch die Rotationsangioplastik entstandene neue Kanal wurde bei 3 Gefäßen mit einem herkömmlichen Ballonkatheter dilatiert (Abb. 2), bei 2 Gefäßen mit einem rotierenden elastischen Drahtelement geweitet (Abb. 3) und bei 3 Gefäßen belassen.

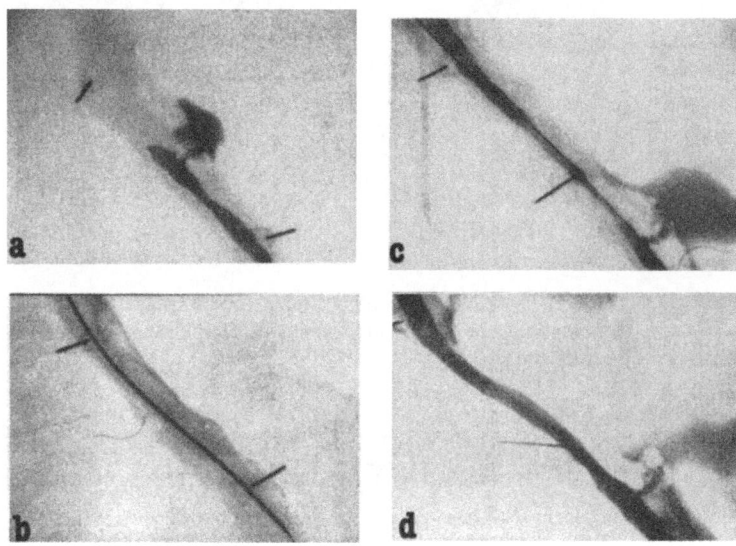

Abb. 2. a Verschlossene A. femoralis sup.; **b** die Rotationswelle hat den Verschluß passiert; **c** Angiographie bei liegendem Wechseldraht: man erkennt den neuen Kanal; **d** Kontrolle nach Ballondilatation

Sonderdruck aus Z Kardiologie, 76: 608–611, 1987, Springer Berlin Heidelberg

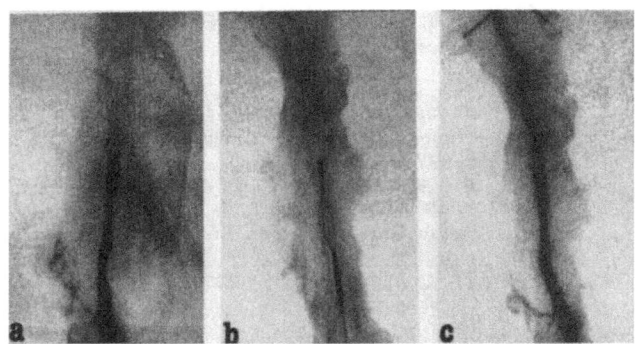

Abb. 3. a Verschlossene A. femoralis sup.; **b** nach Eröffnung des Verschlusses mit der Rotationswelle wird der Kanal mit einem elastischen Drahtelement rotierend geweitet **c** Kontrolle nach Dehnung

In der histologischen Aufarbeitung von 4 Arterien ergaben sich keine Perforationen durch die Rotationswelle. In einem Fall war nach Benutzung eines zu groß dimensionierten Ballonkatheters eine Ruptur der Media zu erkennen.

Der neu entstandene Kanal erschien relativ glatt konturiert (Abb. 4).

Mit Hilfe eines 1,5-mm-Edwards-Angioskops konnten bei 2 Arterien der Verschluß sowie der neu entstandene Kanal optisch dargestellt werden. Auch hier erschienen die Konturen überraschend glatt (Abb. 5).

Diskussion

Chronische arterielle Verschlüsse sind, abhängig von der Verschlußstrecke und Verschlußdauer, nur in etwa 50% der koronaren und der peripheren Gefäße erfolgreich wieder zu eröffnen [9, 13]. Die Rezidivgefahr nach der Eröffnung ist gegenüber der Dehnung einer Stenose in beiden Bereichen deutlich höher.

Die Gefahr der Dissektion und Wandperforation ist stark erhöht, zumal häufig atheromatöse Ulzerationen zugrunde liegen.

Das von Kaltenbach 1985 beschriebene Verfahren [6] gestattet die Passage der Verschlußstrecke mit sehr geringer Perforationsgefahr, weil

1. anstelle eines dünnen Drahtes ein relativ weitlumiger Katheter verwendet wird,
2. die Rotation zu einer weitgehenden Aufhebung der Reibung in axialer (Längs-)Richtung führt, wodurch die Vorwärtsbewegung des Katheters leicht zur Spitze übertragen und Widerstände sensitiv wahrgenommen werden und
3. der konstruktive Aufbau des Rotationskatheters eine extreme Flexibilität mit hoher Rotationsstabilität und Druckfestigkeit in axialer Richtung verbindet.

Das Ziel, eine biegsame Welle auf lange Distanz und über Gefäßbiegungen 1:1 drehstabil zu machen, wurde durch die Verwendung vierfacher Spiralwellen aus V_2A-Stahl gelöst. Dichtungsprobleme und Probleme der manuellen Führung eines rotierenden Kathetersystems konnten durch die Entwicklung spezieller Rotationsschleusen und Rotationsadapter behoben werden.

Von den später beschriebenen Hochgeschwindigkeitsrotationstechniken [8, 11] unterscheidet sich unser Verfahren sowohl technisch als auch im Grundkonzept. Während diese mit Rotationsgeschwindigkeiten bis 150 000 U/min und diamantbesetzten Bohrköpfen eine Abrasion des Verschlußmaterials anstreben, handelt es sich bei unserem Verfahren um eine Verdrängung bzw. Kompression und Volumenreduktion durch Flüssigkeitsabpressung [7]. Die Passage der Verschlußstrecke gleicht in ihrem Ablauf einer stumpfen Präparation.

Unsere bisher durchgeführten experimentellen Untersuchungen zeigen, daß mit dieser Technik unter langsamer Rotation bis 200 U/min auch längerstreckige, alte und verkalkte Gefäßverschlüsse erfolgreich wiedereröffnet werden können, ohne daß Perforationen durch den Rotationskatheter entstehen. Auch die in nur einem Fall sichtbare Dissektion entspricht einem sehr niedrigen Prozentsatz.

Entscheidend ist, daß die Rotationswelle den weichsten Teil des Verschlußkanales findet, in dem sich der letztlich verschließende Thrombus dem arteriosklerotischen Plaque auflagerte. Dieser „hinkt" im Grad der Verhärtung durch Fibrosierung und Verkalkung den Wandanteilen nach. Mit anderen Worten: das Härteste ist die Wand, das Weichste die letzte Verschlußstelle im Restlumen.

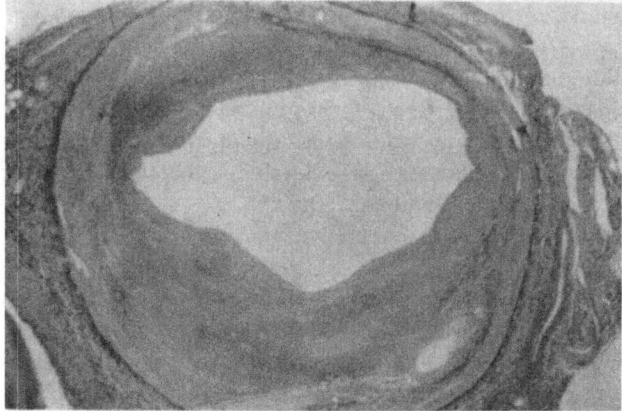

Abb. 4. Die Histologie zeigt eine relativ glatte Oberfläche des neu entstandenen Kanals

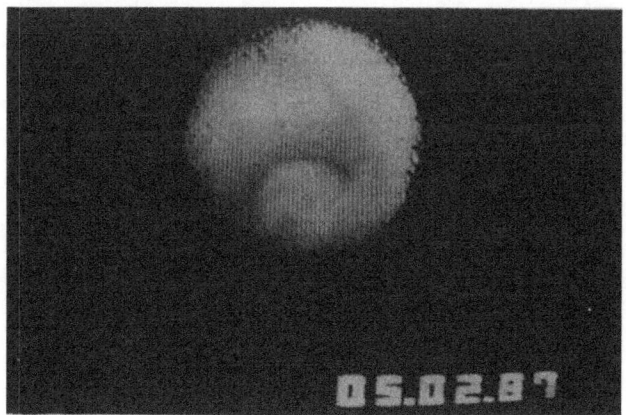

Abb. 5. Angioskopische Darstellung eines glatt berandeten, schlitzförmigen Kanals

14   C. Vallbracht et al.   Sonderdruck aus Z Kardiologie, 76: 608–611, 1987, Springer Berlin Heidelberg

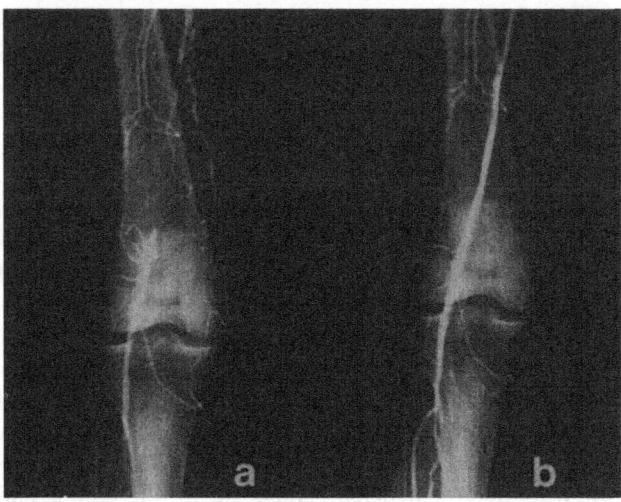

Abb. 6. Patient Nr. 2. **a** 8 cm langer Verschluß der A. fem. sup.; **b** nach Wiedereröffnung mit der Rotationswelle und anschließender Ballondilatation

Seit Dezember 1986 wurde die Technik auch klinisch bei Patienten mit Verschlüssen der Arteria femoralis superficialis und Arteria poplitea angewandt. Die Verschluß-strecken lagen bei 4 Patienten zwischen 4 und 15 cm, die Dauer der Verschlüsse betrug 5 bis 30 Monate. 2 Verschlüsse, darunter der 15 cm lange, konnten erfolgreich wiedereröffnet und danach mit einem Ballonkatheter dilatiert werden. Bei den beiden anderen Patienten, bei denen die herkömmliche Technik versagt hatte, konnten im gleichen Eingriff die vorbestehenden Dissektionswege mit der Rotationswelle nicht umgangen werden. Perforationen oder Dissektionen durch den Rotationskatheter traten in keinem Fall auf (Abb. 6).

Die weitere Erfahrung muß zeigen, ob diese ersten positiven Eindrücke bestätigt werden können. Neben Vorteilen bei peripheren sind solche bei koronaren und renalen Gefäßverschlüssen zu erwarten.

Ob die Weitung mittels langsam rotierender und expandierender Drahtelemente Vorteile gegenüber der herkömmlichen Ballondehnung erbringt, muß abgewartet werden.

Literatur

1. Bussmann W-D, Grützmacher P, Faßbinder W, Ruminski J, Meyer P, Schoeppe W, Kaltenbach M (1984) Transluminale Angioplastie von Nierenarterienstenosen: Langzeitergebnisse. Verh Dtsch Ges f Inn Med 90: 77–757
2. Dotter CT, Judkins MP (1964) Transluminal treatment of arteriosclerotic obstruction: Description of a new technique and a preliminary report of its application. Circulation 30: 654
3. Faxon DP, Kelsey S, Kellett MA, Ryan TJ, Detre K and members of the NHLBI PTCA Registry (1986) Predictors of a successful angioplasty (NHLBI-PTCA registry). Circulation 74, Suppl II: 768
4. Grüntzig A, Myler R, Hanna E, Turina M (1977) Transluminal angioplasty of coronary artery stenoses. Circulation 84: 56–66 (Suppl.)
5. Grüntzig A, Hopff H (1974) Perkutane Rekanalisation chronischer arterieller Verschlüsse mit einem neuen Dilatationskatheter. Modifikation der Dottertechnik. Dtsch Med Wschr 99: 2502–2510
6. Kaltenbach M DE 3532653 A 1, P 3532653.o 13.9.1985
7. Kaltenbach M, Beyer J, Walter S, Klepzig H, Schmidts L (1984) Prolonged application of pressure in transluminal coronary angioplasty. Cath and Cardiovasc Diagn 10: 213–219
8. Kensey K, Nash J, Abrahams C, Lake K, Zarins CK (1986) Recanalization of obstructed arteries using a flexible rotating tip catheter. Circulation, Vol. 74, Suppl II: 1821
9. Kober G, Vallbracht C, Lang H, Bussmann W-D, Hopf R, Kunkel B, Kaltenbach M (1985) Transluminale koronare Angioplastik 1977–1985. Erfahrungen bei 1000 Eingriffen. Radiologe 25: 346
10. Mathias K, Gospos CH, Thron A et al (1980) Percutaneous transluminal treatment of supraaortic artery obstruction. Ann Radiol 23: 281
11. Ritchie JL, Hansen DD, Vracko H, Auth D (1986) In vivo rotational thrombectomy evaluation by angioscopy. Circulation Vol 74, Suppl II: 1822
12. Simpson JB, Blaim DS, Robert E, Harrison DC (1982) A new catheter system for coronary angioplasty. Am J Cardiol 49: 1216–1222
13. Zeitler E (1985) Die perkutane transluminale Rekanalisation chronischer Stenosen und Verschlüsse peripherer Arterien. Wien Med Wschr 135: 384–392

Eingegangen 24. Juni 1987
akzeptiert 3. Juli 1987

Für die Verfasser:
Dr. med. C. Vallbracht, Zentrum der Inneren Medizin, Abt. für Kardiologie, Klinikum der Universität, Theodor-Stern-Kai 7, 6000 Frankfurt/Main

Rotationsangioplastik – Erste klinische Ergebnisse bei peripheren Gefäßverschlüssen

C. Vallbracht, M. Schweitzer, J. Kress, W. Bamberg, J. Kollath, D. Liermann,
C. Paasch, K. Rauber, F. J. Roth, J. Prignitz, W. Beinborn, H. Landgraf,
H. K. Breddin, W. Schoop und M. Kaltenbach

Low speed rotational angioplasty- preliminary clinical results in chronic peripheral occlusions

Summary: After experimental investigations in post-mortem human arteries, 19 patients with chronic peripheral artery occlusions were treated with a new technique between December 1986 and October 1987. In 17 patients the superficial femoral artery, and in two patients the popliteal artery, was completely occluded. The length of occlusions were between 5 and 25 cm (mean 10.9 cm); the duration (estimated according to patient's history) was 5–48 months (mean 17.2 months). In five patients, durations of up to 30 months had been documented by angiography.

A flexible, blunt, motor-driven rotating catheter was introduced over an 8 or 9 F sheet and rotational angioplasty was performed at low speed, up to 200 rpm. In 11/14 patients in whom this new technique was used as the first attempt, the occlusions could be successfully reopened. In two patients after failure of the conventional technique the rotating catheter could not bypass the preexisting dissections in the same intervention. In 2/3 further patients after failure of the conventional technique the occlusions could be successfully reopened in a second intervention after several weeks.

In none of our 19 patients did a perforation occur. It is concluded that by using the new technique, chronic peripheral artery occlusions can be reopened with a high success rate and without the danger of vessel wall perforation. The method can also be applied in patients in whom conventional techniques have failed.

Zusammenfassung: Nach experimentellen Vorarbeiten wurde im Zeitraum von Dezember 1986 bis Oktober 1987 bei 19 Patienten mit langstreckigen Verschlüssen peripherer Arterien eine neue Technik zur Wiedereröffnung eingesetzt. Bei 17 Patienten war die A. femoralis sup. und bei 2 Patienten die A. poplitea komplett verschlossen. Die Verschlußlängen lagen zwischen 5 und 25 cm ($\bar{x}$: 10.9 cm); die Verschlußdauer betrug nach anamnestischen Angaben 5–48 Monate ($\bar{x}$: 17,2 Monate) und war bei 5 Patienten angiographisch dokumentiert (längste ang. Verschlußdauer: 30 Monate). Über eine 8F- oder 9F-Schleuse wurde ein elektrisch angetriebener, flexibler, stumpfer Rotationskatheter eingeführt und die Verschlußstrecke mit Rotationsgeschwindigkeiten bis 200 U/min passiert. Bei 11/14 primär mit dieser Technik behandelten Patienten konnten die Verschlüsse erfolgreich eröffnet und anschließend mit einem Ballonkatheter dilatiert werden. Nach erfolglosem Versuch mit der herkömmlichen Technik konnten im gleichen Eingriff bei 2/2 Patienten die hierbei entstandenen Dissektionswege nicht umgangen werden; bei 2/3 weiteren Patienten nach erfolglosem konventionellem Versuch konnte in einem zweiten Eingriff nach mehreren Wochen die neue Technik die Verschlüsse eröffnen.

Perforationen traten in keinem Fall auf. Es wird gefolgert, daß die neue Technik chronische periphere Gefäßverschlüsse vergleichsweise schonend wiedereröffnen kann und auch für bisher nicht behandelbare Obstruktionen in Betracht kommt.

Einleitung

Die Grenzen der nichtoperativen Erweiterung arteriosklerotisch verengter Blutgefäße unterschiedlicher Lokalisationen mit der heute weltweit eingeführten Technik der Ballondilatation nach Grüntzig [3] liegen bei hochgradigen, mit dem Führungsdraht oder Ballonkatheter nicht zu passierenden Stenosen und insbesondere bei kompletten Gefäßverschlüssen.

Abhängig von Verschlußdauer und -länge sowie dem Nachweis von Gefäßverkalkungen werden für periphere [16] und subakute koronare [8, 9, 11] Gefäßverschlüsse Akuterfolgsraten von nur etwa 50–80% angegeben.

Seit der Erstbeschreibung eines speziellen Rotationskatheters durch Kaltenbach 1985 [4] haben wir gemeinsam an der Fortentwicklung dieser neuen Technik gearbeitet, bei der eine langsam rotierende Welle benutzt wird [6]. In experimentellen Untersuchungen an menschlichen Leichenarterien [14] zeigte sich die Möglichkeit, hiermit auch alte und verkalkte Gefäßverschlüsse wiederzueröffnen, bei denen die herkömmliche Technik versagte.

Perforationen wurden nicht beobachtet, histologische und angioskopische Kontrollen des neu entstandenen Kanals zeigten eine relativ glatte Oberfläche.

Aufgrund dieser ermutigenden Ergebnisse begannen wir im Dezember 1986 mit der klinischen Anwendung bei Patienten mit peripheren Gefäßverschlüssen [15]. Im folgenden soll über die ersten 19 Patienten berichtet werden.

Key words: rotational angioplasty; peripheral occlusion

Schlüsselwörter: Rotationsangioplastik; periphere Gefäßverschlüsse

Sonderdruck aus Z Kardiologie, 77: 352–357, 1988, Springer Berlin Heidelberg

Patienten

Im Zeitraum von Dezember 1986 bis Oktober 1987 wurden 19 Patienten mit der neuen Technik behandelt. Es waren 6 Frauen und 13 Männer im Alter von 35 bis 81 Jahren. Bei 17 Patienten war die A. femoralis superficialis und bei 2 Patienten die A. poplitea komplett verschlossen.

Klinische und angiographische Befunde

Klinisch waren vor Behandlung 15 Patienten im Stadium II nach Fontaine; die schmerzfreie Gehstrecke lag zwischen 30 und 300 m ($\overline{x}$: 125 m). 4 Patienten waren im Stadium IV und klagten über Ruheschmerz.

In den Doppler-Druckmessungen vor Behandlung lag der Bein-/Arm-Quotient [12] zwischen 0,29 und 0,86 ($\overline{x}$: 0,53).

Die Verschlußdauer betrug nach anamnestischen Angaben 5 bis 48 Monate (im Mittel 17,2 Monate). Bei 5 Patienten lagen angiographische Voruntersuchungen vor; der angiographisch dokumentierte Verschluß lag in diesen Fällen 6, 18, 18, 24 und 30 Monate zurück.

Die Verschlußlänge lag zwischen 5 und 25 cm (im Mittel bei 10,9 cm). Bei 13/19 Patienten bestanden deutliche Gefäßverkalkungen (vgl. Tab. 1–3).

11 Patienten wurden zusammen mit dem Zentrum für Radiologie (Leiter: Prof. Dr. J. Kollath) und der Abteilung für Angiologie (Leiter: Prof. Dr. H. K. Breddin) der Universität Frankfurt behandelt, 8 Patienten zusammen mit der Abteilung für Radiologie (Leiter: Prof. Dr. F. J. Roth) und der Abteilung für Innere Medizin und Angiologie (Leiter: Prof. Dr. W. Schoop) der Aggertalklinik der LVA in Engelskirchen.

Technik und Untersuchungsablauf

Nach lokaler Betäubung wurde die A. femoralis antegrad punktiert und über einen 5F-Katheter zunächst eine konventionelle angiographische Darstellung der gesamten Extremität durchgeführt. Anhand dieser Aufnahmen wurde die Verschlußlänge gemessen und zur Korrektur des Vergrößerungsfaktors auf die bekannte Weite des Angiographiekatheters bezogen.

Über einen Wechseldraht wurde dann eine 8F- oder 9F-Schleuse mit Luer-Anschluß eingelegt. Die unterschied-

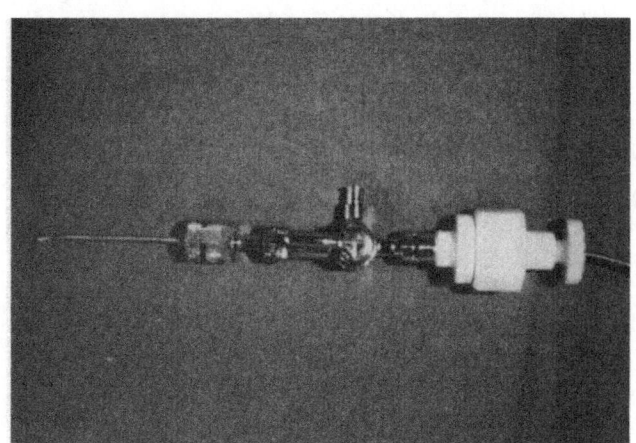

Abb. 1. Rotationsschleuse

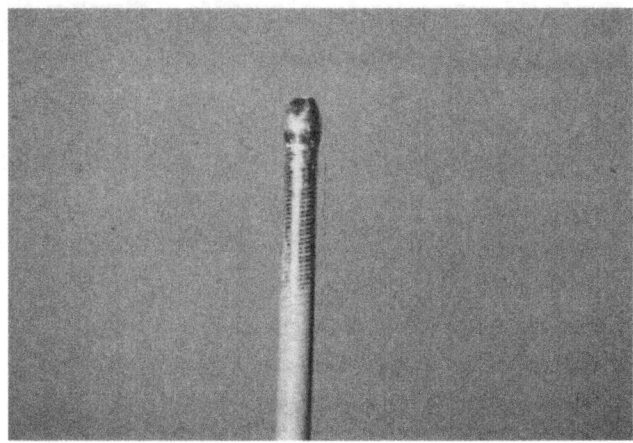

Abb 2. Rotationskatheter aus $4 \times 0{,}2$-mm-V2A-Spiraldrähten mit stumpfem Kopf und Teflonüberzug

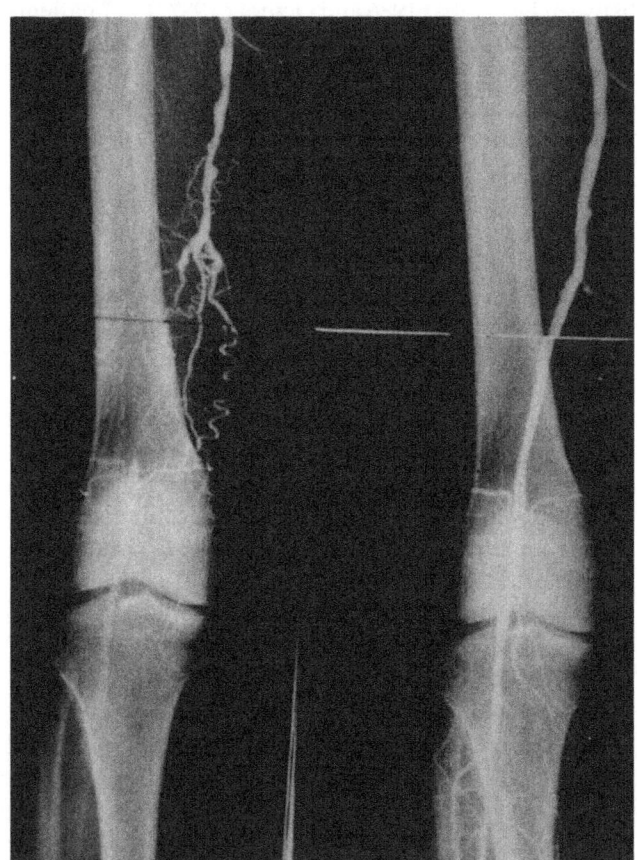

Abb. 3. A. femoralis sup. mit mehreren Stenosen bis 60% Lumeneinengung im proximalen und einem 10,4 cm langen kompletten Verschluß im distalen Abschnitt. Links vor, rechts nach Rotationsangioplastik und Ballondilatation (Patient L. F.)

lich langen Schleusen wurden bis auf etwa 5 cm an die Verschlußstelle herangeschoben. Mittels digitaler Substraktionsangiographie wurde ein Standbild angefertigt, das dem Durchleuchtungsbild unterlegt werden konnte (sog. Road-Mapping).

Nach Gabe von 5000 E Heparin intraarteriell wurde eine spezielle Rotationsschleuse auf den Luer-Ansatz geschraubt (Abb. 1) und das System über den Seitenschluß für den Untersuchungszeitraum mit einer Kombination

Tabelle 1. Rotationsangioplastik als Ersteingriff

Patient	Verschluß			Kalk	Komplikationen	Ergebnis
	Lokalisation	Dauer (Monate)	Länge (cm)			
B. G., m.	A. fem. sup.	8	20,6	++	–	+
T. H., w.	A. fem. sup.	7	9,5	+	–	+
D. O., m.	A. fem. sup.	18 (angio.)	16	++	Hämatom ing.	–
C. J., w.	A. fem. sup./A. poplitea	30	10	+++	–	–
G. M., w.	A. fem. sup./A. poplitea	6 (angio.)	25	+++	–	+
H. E., w.	A. fem. sup.	8	7,1	++	–	+
L. F., m.	A. fem. sup.	6	10,4	++	–	+
S. W., m.	A. fem. sup.	12	5	–	–	+
W. F., m.	A. fem. sup.	12	15	++	Dissektion (folgenlos)	–
K. J., m.	A. fem. sup.	12	6	–	–	+
S. L., m.	A. fem. sup.	18	12	–	–	+
W. F., w.	A. poplitea	48 (gesch.) 30 (angio.)	8	+	–	+
B. A., m.	A. fem. sup.	30	12	+	–	+
S. U., m.	A. fem. sup.	48 (gesch.) 18 (angio.)	12	+	–	+

aus 2000 E Heparin/h und 100 000 E Urokinase/h perfundiert. Durch die Rotationsschleuse, die die freie Drehung des Katheters bei dichtem Gefäßabschluß ermöglicht, wurde nun der Rotationskatheter aus 4-Polyolefin-überschrumpften V2A-Spiraldrähten [6] mit rundem Kopf eingeführt (Abb. 2).

Bei Erreichen des Verschlusses wurde über einen Fußschalter der angeschlossene Elektromotor gestartet und die Verschlußstrecke mit Rotationsgeschwindigkeiten von 100–200 U/min passiert.

Nach Erreichen des peripheren Anschlusses wurde zunächst Kontrastmittel über den Rotationskatheter injiziert, um die korrekte Lage im Gefäßlumen zu dokumentieren. Danach wurde ein Wechseldraht durch den Rotationskatheter eingeführt. Nach Plazierung im peripheren Gefäßabschnitt wurde der Rotationskatheter zurückgezogen, der entstandene neue Kanal bei liegendem Wechseldraht angiographisch dargestellt und anschließend mit einem herkömmlichen Ballonkatheter dilatiert (Abb. 3–5).

Nach einer abschließenden Angiographie der gesamten Extremität wurde die Schleuse entfernt und nach manueller Kompression ein Druckverband für 24 Stunden angelegt.

Alle Patienten erhielten mindestens eine Woche vor, während und für die Zeit nach dem Eingriff Acetylsalicylsäure 1,5 g/Tag [1]. Unmittelbar nach dem Eingriff wurde für mindestens 24 Stunden eine kontrollierte intravenöse Heparinisierung mit 1000–1200 E/Stunde angeschlossen.

Ergebnisse

a) Angiographische Ergebnisse
1. Bei 11 von 14 Patienten, bei denen diese Technik als Ersteingriff angewandt wurde, konnten die Verschlüsse von bis zu 25 cm Länge und bis zu 30 Monaten angiographisch dokumentierter Dauer erfolgreich wiedereröffnet werden (Abb. 3 und 4).

Bei 2 Patienten waren die Verschlußstrecken von 15 bzw. 16 cm mit Verschlußzeiten von mindestens 12 bzw. 18 Monaten und ausgeprägten Verkalkungen nicht zu passieren.

Bei einer Patientin mußte der Eingriff nach 50 Minuten wegen allgemeiner Unruhe abgebrochen werden (Tab. 1).

2. Bei 2 Patienten, bei denen die herkömmliche Technik versagt und zu einer Dissektion geführt hatte, konnte der

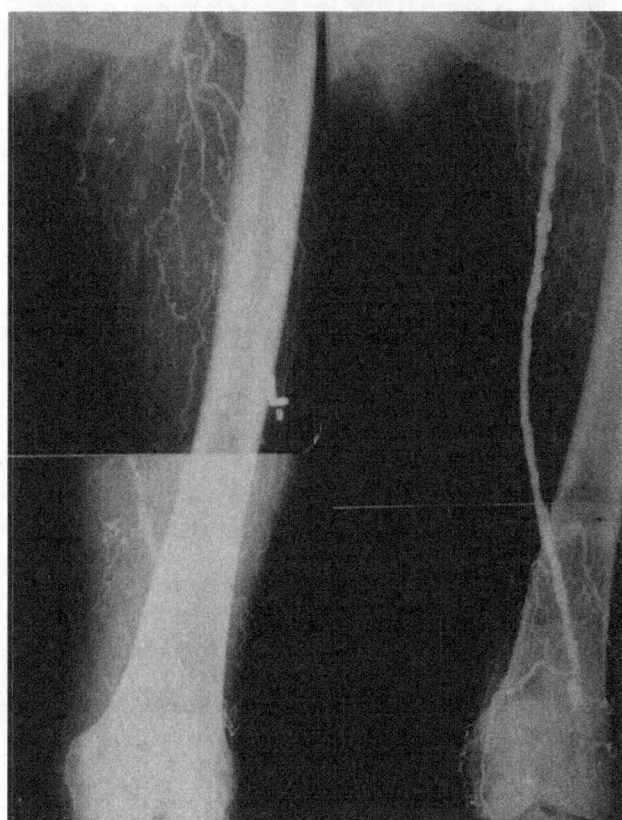

Abb. 4. 25 cm langer, stark verkalkter Verschluß der A. femoralis sup. bei einer 78jährigen Diabetikerin. Links vor, rechts nach Rotationsangioplastik und Ballondilatation (Patientin G. M.)

Tabelle 2. Rotationsangioplastik nach erfolglosem konventionellem Versuch der Wiedereröffnung (gleicher Eingriff)

Patient	Verschluß			Kalk	Komplikation	Ergebnis
	Lokalisation	Dauer (Monate)	Länge (cm)			
C. O., m.	A. fem. sup.	24 (angio.)	9	+	–	–
B. B., w.	A. poplitea	5	6	+++	–	–

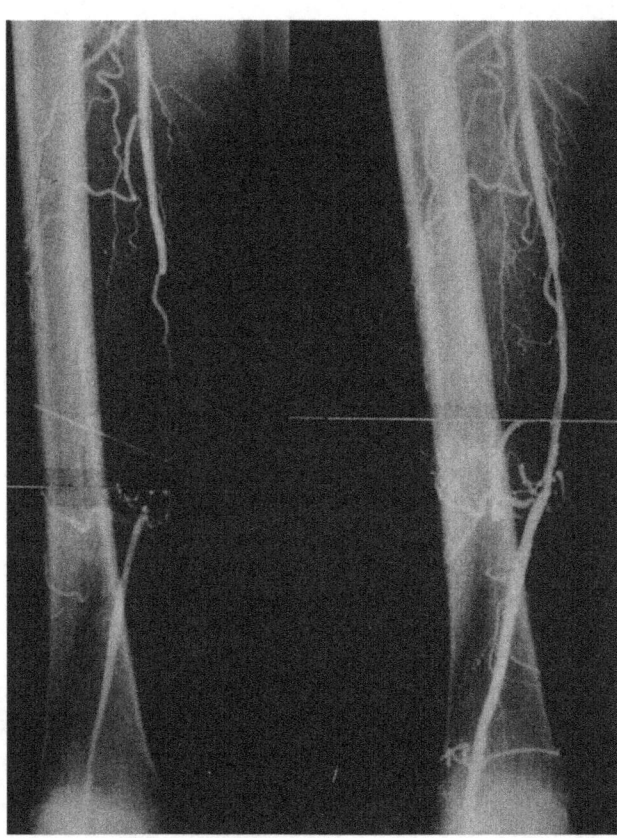

Abb. 5. 11 cm langer Verschluß der A. femoralis sup., der mit der konventionellen Technik nicht zu eröffnen war. Links vor, rechts nach Rotationsangioplastik und Ballondilatation (Patient G. O.)

Rotationskatheter *im gleichen Eingriff* die bestehenden Dissektionswege nicht umgehen (Tab. 2).
3. Bei 3 weiteren Patienten war ebenfalls eine Wiedereröffnung mit der konventionellen Technik erfolglos geblieben. 4 Wochen bzw. 4 Monate nach diesem ersten Eingriff konnten bei 2 von 3 Patienten diese Verschlüsse mit dem Rotationskatheter erfolgreich wiedereröffnet werden (Abb. 5).

Bei der dritten Patientin mit einem kurzstreckigen Verschluß der A. fem. sup. fehlte ein eigentlicher Gefäßstummel, so daß der Rotationskatheter – wie zuvor auch der konventionelle Führungsdraht – immer wieder in die dort abgehende sehr kräftige Kollaterale abwich (Tab. 3).

b) Funktionelle Ergebnisse
Unter den 13 erfolgreich behandelten Patienten war nach dem Eingriff bei 8 die Gehstrecke nicht mehr durch eine Claudicatio begrenzt.
Ein Patient war nach 200 m jetzt durch seine Angina pectoris bei koronarer Dreigefäßkrankheit limitiert.
Bei einer 78jährigen, inoperablen Diabetikerin konnte durch die Wiedereröffnung der A. femoralis superficialis (25 cm) bei weiterhin verschlossener A. poplitea eine Gehstrecke von 300 m (zuvor Ruheschmerz) erreicht werden, die Nekrose der Fußzehen heilte zusehends.
Bei einer Patientin kam es trotz gutem angiographischem Akutergebnis nicht zu einer funktionellen Verbesserung. Die Kontrollangiographie nach 2 Tagen ergab einen Reverschluß, möglicherweise bedingt durch eine fehlende Heparinisierung nach dem Eingriff. Bei 2 Patienten stehen funktionelle Kontrollen noch aus.
Der Bein-/Arm-Quotient verbesserte sich bei 11 Patienten von im Mittel 0,55 auf im Mittel 0,86 (Tab. 4).

c) Komplikationen
Gefäßperforationen traten in keinem Fall auf. Bei einem Patienten mit einem 15 cm langen und stark verkalkten Verschluß kam es zu einer folgenlosen Dissektion.
Einmal trat eine größere Nachblutung an der Punktionsstelle auf, die ohne weitere Probleme gestillt werden konnte.
Bei einem Patienten war eine kleine periphere Embolie nachweisbar, die klinisch stumm blieb und in der Kontrolluntersuchung nach 2 Monaten nicht mehr bestand.

Geplante Nachuntersuchungen
Alle Patienten wurden systematisch weiter beobachtet.

Tabelle 3. Rotationsangioplastik nach erfolglosem konventionellem Versuch der Wiedereröffnung (Zweiteingriff mit Mindestabstand 4 Wochen)

Patient	Verschluß			Kalk	Komplikation	Ergebnis
	Lokalisation	Dauer (Monate)	Länge (cm)			
G. O., m.	A. fem. sup.	7	11	–	–	+
G. C., m.	A. fem. sup.	12	12	–	–	+
B. A., w.	A. fem. sup.	15	1	–	–	–

Tabelle 4. Funktionelle Ergebnisse

Patient	vor Wiedereröffnung		nach Wiedereröffnung		Anmerkungen
	Gehstrecke (m)	Bein-/Arm-Doppler-Quotient	Gehstrecke (m)	Bein-/Arm-Doppler-Quotient	
B. G., m.	150	0,38	?	0,75	Angina pectoris nach 200 m
T. H., w.	100	0,53	100	0,55	Angio:Reverschluß
G. M., w.	Ruheschmerz	0,30	300	0,60	A. poplitea weiter verschlossen
H. E., w.	150	0,70	unbegrenzt	0,97	–
L. F., m.	150	0,72	unbegrenzt	1,1	–
S. W., m.	200	0,64	unbegrenzt	0,92	–
K. J., m.	30	0,32	steht aus	steht aus	–
S. L., m.	100	0,69	unbegrenzt	1,05	–
W. F., w.	200	0,37	unbegrenzt	0,82	–
B. A., m.	100	0,29	steht aus	steht aus	–
S. U., m.	300	0,86	unbegrenzt	1,0	–
G. O., m.	50	0,65	unbegrenzt	0,79	–
G. C., m.	100	0,50	unbegrenzt	0,86	–

Eine angiographische und funktionelle Kontrolluntersuchung ist nach 6 Monaten vorgesehen.

Diskussion

Arteriosklerotischen Gefäßverschlüssen liegen oft ulzerös veränderte Atherombeete zugrunde; die Gefahr, bei dem Versuch der Wiedereröffnung eine Dissektion zu erzeugen bzw. das Gefäßlumen zu verlassen, ist in diesen Fällen deutlich erhöht und nimmt mit steigender Verschlußlänge zu.

Ein relativ dünner Draht, wie er üblicherweise bei der konventionellen Technik zur Wiedereröffnung benutzt wird, birgt dabei offensichtlich ein höheres Risiko als der hier verwendete flexible Katheter hoher Drehsteifigkeit mit großem Außendurchmesser von 2 mm und stumpfem Kopf [6].

Die langsame Drehung unter geringem axialem Druck bewirkt, daß der Rotationskatheter den Weg des geringsten Widerstandes sucht. Während die Gefäßwand hart und zum Teil verkalkt ist, stellt der letztlich verschließende Thrombus den weichsten Teil des Verschlußquerschnittes dar, der in seiner Verhärtung durch Fibrosierung den anderen Strukturen sehr lange Zeit (bis zu mehreren Jahren) nachhinken kann. Dies mag erklären, warum auch bei nachweislich mehr als 30 Monaten Verschlußdauer noch eine Wiedereröffnung gelang.

Der Mechanismus der Wiedereröffnung geht im Gegensatz zu beschriebenen Hochgeschwindigkeitsrotationstechniken [7, 10] nicht mit einer Abrasion von Verschlußmaterial einher, ist also mit einem Bohrvorgang im eigentlichen Sinne nicht zu vergleichen. Vielmehr wird ein neuer Gefäßkanal geschaffen, ohne daß thrombotisches oder arteriosklerotisches Material nach proximal oder distal verschleppt wird. Der pathophysiologische Grundvorgang ist, wie für die Druckanwendung allgemein früher beschrieben [5], eine Volumenverkleinerung durch Flüssigkeitsabpressung aus dem atheromatösen Gewebe.

Unsere ersten klinischen Erfahrungen mit dieser neuen Technik zeigen, daß selbst langstreckige Verschlüsse mit zum Teil starker Verkalkung der Arterienwand erfolgreich rekanalisiert werden können, bei denen mit der herkömmlichen Technik oft Probleme bestehen [16]. Auch nach erfolglosem konventionellem Versuch der Wiedereröffnung kann die Rotationsangioplastik mit Aussicht auf Erfolg eingesetzt werden; der Eingriff sollte dann allerdings im zeitlichen Mindestabstand von einigen Wochen erfolgen. Dieser Zeitraum ist erforderlich, um durch den Ersteingriff entstandene Dissektionswege verheilen zu lassen.

Wie in den experimentellen Untersuchungen [14] erwies sich die neue Technik auch in den bisher durchgeführten klinischen Eingriffen als wenig traumatisch. Gefäßperforationen oder andere schwerwiegende Komplikationen traten in keinem Fall auf. Hierin scheint uns ein wesentlicher Vorteil sowohl gegenüber den konventionellen als auch gegenüber anderen neuen Verfahren wie den Hochgeschwindigkeitstechniken [7, 10] zu liegen.

Es ist denkbar, daß der schonende Vorgang der Eröffnung des ursprünglichen Gefäßlumens auch einen positiven Einfluß auf die Langzeitergebnisse hat, die bisher insbesondere bei langstreckigen Verschlüssen enttäuschend waren [2]. Langzeitbeobachtungen mit funktionellen und angiographischen Kontrollen aller behandelten Patienten sind vorgesehen.

Die günstigen Erfahrungen an peripheren Arterien lassen die Anwendbarkeit der Methode in anderen Gefäßgebieten erwarten; entsprechende Untersuchungen mit Modifikationen der Technik wurden begonnen.

Nachtrag bei der Korrektur

Bis Mai 1988 wurden insgesamt 43 Patienten mit der neuen Technik behandelt.

Bei Ersteingriff und Verschlußlängen unter 10 cm betrug die Akuterfolgsrate 8/8; bei Verschlußlängen über 10 cm (längster Verschluß 30 cm) konnten 16/20 erfolgreich rekanalisiert werden.

Nach erfolglosem Versuch der Wiedereröffnung mit der konventionellen Technik wurden bisher 15 Patienten behandelt. Dabei konnte bei einem zeitlichen Abstand zum Ersteingriff von weniger als 4 Wochen kein Erfolg erzielt werden (4 Patienten). Bei einem Abstand von mehr als 4 Wochen (11 Patienten) konnte bei 7/11 eine erfolgreiche Rekanalisation erreicht werden.

Perforationen oder andere ernste Komplikationen sind weiterhin nicht aufgetreten. Inzwischen wurde die Indikation auf Verschlüsse der A. iliaca ausgedehnt.

Literatur

1. Breddin HK (1982) Treatment with platelet function inhibitors. In: Kaltenbach M, Grüntzig A, Rentrop K, Bussmann WD (eds) Transluminal coronary angioplasty and intracoronary thrombolysis. Springer-Verlag, Heidelberg New York, pp 41–43

2. Gallino A, Mahler F, Probst P, Nachbur B (1984) Percutaneous transluminal angioplasty of the arteries of the lower limbs: a 5 year follow-up. Circulation, Vol 70, No 4: 619–623

3. Grüntzig A, Hopff H (1974) Perkutane Rekanalisation chronischer arterieller Verschlüsse mit einem neuen Dilatationskatheter. Modifikation der Dottertechnik. Dtsch Med Wschr 99: 2502–2510

4. Kaltenbach M (1985) DE 3532653 A 1, P 3532653, 13. 9. 1985

5. Kaltenbach M, Beyer J, Klepzig H, Schmidts L, Hübner K (1982) Effect of 5 kg/cm² pressure on atherosclerotic vessel wall segments. In: Kaltenbach M, Grüntzig A, Rentrop K, Bussmann WD (eds) Transluminal coronary angioplasty and intracoronary thrombolysis. Springer-Verlag, Heidelberg New Yor

6. Kaltenbach M, Vallbracht C (1987) Rotationsangioplastik – ein neues Katheterverfahren. Fortschr Med 105 Jg Nr 21: 412–414

7. Kensey K, Nash J, Abrahams C, Lake K, Zarius CK (1986) Recanaliszation of obstructed arteries using a flexible rotating tip catheter. Circulation Vol 74, Suppl II: 1821 (abstr)

8. Kober G, Vallbracht C, Lang H, Bussmann WD, Hopf R, Kunkel B, Kaltenbach M (1985) Transluminale koronare Angioplastik 1977–1985. Erfahrungen bei 1000 Eingriffen. Radiologe 25: 346

9. Meier B, Grüntzig A (1984) Resultate der transluminalen Koronardilatation Dtsch med Wschr 109: 675–677

10. Ritchie JL, Hansen DD, Vracko H, Auth D (1986) In vivo rotational thrombectomy-evaluation by angioscopy. Circulation Vol 74, Suppl II: 1822 (abstr)

11. Savage R, Hollmann J, Grüntzig AR, King SB III, Douglas J, Tankersley R (1982) Can percutaneous transluminal coronary angioplasty be performed in patients with total occlusions? Circulation 66–II: 330 (abstr)

12. Schoop W (1976) Die Ultraschall-Doppler-Methode in der Diagnostik der arteriellen und venösen Störungen in den Extremitäten. Internist 17: 580

13. Thulesius O, Gjöres JE (1971) Use of doppler shift detection for determining peripheral arterial blood pressure. Angiology 22: 594

14. Vallbracht C, Kress J, Schweitzer M, Schneider M, Wendt Th, Ziemen M, Kollath J, Bamberg W, Kaltenbach M (1987) Rotationsangioplastik – ein neues Verfahren zur Gefäßwiedereröffnung und -erweiterung. Experimentelle Befunde. Z Kardiol 76: 608–611

15. Vallbracht C, Schweizer M, Kress J, Kollath J, Bamberg W, Ziemen M, Kaltenbach M (1987) Low speed rotational angioplasty – preliminary clinical results. Circulation Vol 76, Supp IV, III (abstr)

16. Zeitler E (1985) Die perkutane transluminale Rekanalisation chronischer Stenosen und Verschlüsse peripherer Arterien. Wien Med Wschr 135: 384–392

Eingegangen 19. Januar 1988
akzeptiert 24. März 1988

Für die Verfasser:
Dr. med. C. Vallbracht, Abt. f. Kardiologie, Zentrum der Inneren Medizin, Universität Frankfurt, Theodor-Stern-Kai 7, 6000 Frankfurt 70

Rotationsangioplastik – Wiedereröffnung chronischer Arterienverschlüsse mit einem langsam rotierenden Katheter

Klinische Ergebnisse bei 100 Patienten

C. Vallbracht, D. Liermann, I. Prignitz, B. Süss, H. Awiszus, C. Paasch,
H. Landgraf, W. Beinborn, G. Stickelmann, J. Kollath, F. J. Roth, W. Schoop,
H. K. Breddin und M. Kaltenbach

Zusammenfassung. Von Dezember 1986 bis Januar 1989 wurden 100 Patienten mit chronischen Verschlüssen peripherer Arterien mit der neuen Technik der Rotationsangioplastik behandelt, die zur Wiedereröffnung einen relativ dicken, flexiblen und stumpfen Katheter benutzt, der von einem Elektromotor angetrieben wird (100–200 U/min). Bei Ersteingriff lag die Akuterfolgsrate bei der A. femoralis superficialis/A. poplitea bei Verschlußlängen unter 10 cm über 90%, bei Verschlüssen über 10 cm noch bei 80%. Nach erfolglosem Versuch mit konventionellen Techniken konnten noch 65% der Verschlüsse erfolgreich wiedereröffnet werden. Bei 7 von 12 Patienten mit Verschlüssen der A. iliaca gelang die Rekanalisation. Perforationen oder andere schwerwiegende Komplikationen traten nicht auf. Es wird gefolgert, daß das neue Verfahren besonders effektiv und schonend chronische Gefäßverschlüsse wiedereröffnen kann und auch bei solchen Obstruktionen in Betracht kommt, die bisher ohne Operation nicht zu behandeln waren.

Low speed rotational angioplasty – recanalisation of chronically occluded arteries with a slowly rotating catheter

Summary. Between December 1986 and January 1989, 100 patients with chronic occlusions of peripheral arteries were treated with the new technique of low speed rotational angioplasty. This uses a relatively thick, flexible and blunt catheter, which is driven by an electric motor (100 to 200 r.p.m.). The success rate in the superficial femoral and popliteal arteries at the initial intervention for occlusions less than 10 cm was 90%, for occlusions of less than 10 cm, it was 80%. Occlusions on which conventional techniques had failed were successfully recanalised in 65%. Recanalisation was also successful in seven out of 12 patients with occluded iliac arteries. There were no perforations or other serious complications. It is concluded that the new method is particularly effective and safe for recanalisation of chronic vascular occlusions and should also be considered for cases which previously could only be treated surgically.

* Hersteller: Dr. Ing. Osypka, Basler Straße 109, 7889 Grenzach-Wyhlen

Einleitung

Die nichtoperative Erweiterung arteriosklerotisch verengter Blutgefäße, von Charles T. Dotter 1964 erstmals an peripheren Arterien durchgeführt [2] und von Andreas Grüntzig mit der Einführung der Ballondilatation entscheidend weiterentwickelt [5], gehört heute zur klinischen Routine vieler Zentren in der ganzen Welt. Neben Arterien der unteren Extremität [5, 15] spielen besonders Koronarstenosen [9] und Stenosen der Nierenarterien eine wesentliche Rolle. Durch vielfältige technische Verbesserungen wie die Einführung steuerbarer Ballonkatheter [12] können heute mehr als 90% aller angegangenen Arterienverengungen erfolgreich erweitert werden [3, 9].

Die heutige Grenze der Methode liegt bei kompletten Gefäßverschlüssen; periphere Gefäßverschlüsse von mehr als 10 cm Länge und subakute Koronararterienverschlüsse sind bisher nur in etwa 50–60% der Fälle erfolgreich wiederzueröffnen [9, 15], wobei mit zunehmender Verschlußdauer und nachweisbaren Gefäßverkalkungen die Chance der Rekanalisation weiter sinkt. Chronische Verschlüsse der A. iliaca gelten aufgrund unbefriedigender Akutergebnisse (30–40% Akuterfolg) und relativ häufiger Komplikationen (Dissektionen, Embolien) bisher allgemein nicht als Indikation zur Angioplastik und werden operativ behandelt [4].

Wir haben in Frankfurt seit 1984 an der Entwicklung einer neuen Technik gearbeitet, bei der eine langsam rotie-

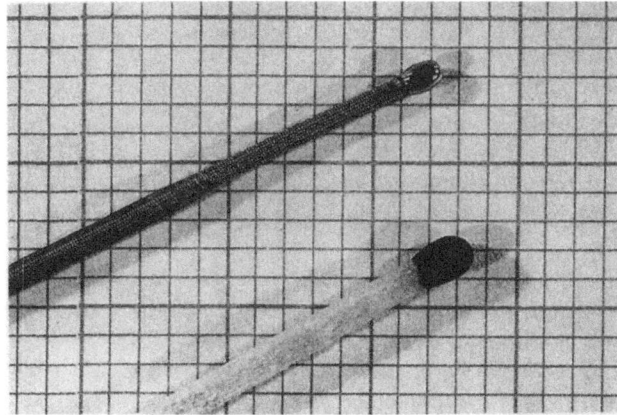

Abb. 1. Rotationskatheter aus 4 × 0,2 mm V₂A-Stahldrähten mit Teflonschrumpfschlauch und olivenförmigem, stumpfem Kopf (Größenvergleich: Streichholz)

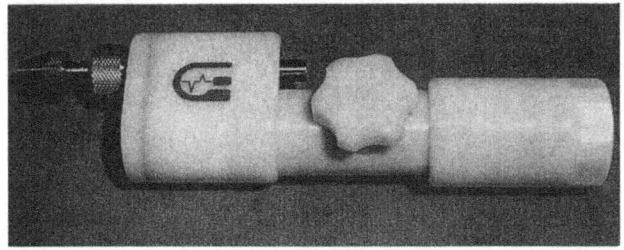

Abb. 2. Elektromotor mit Batterieantrieb. Die 9-V-Batterie wird unter einen sterilen Schraubdeckel eingesetzt

rende, flexible Welle zur Rekanalisation benutzt wird [6, 13, 14]. Experimentelle Untersuchungen an menschlichen Leichenarterien zeigten, daß hiermit auch alte und verkalkte Gefäßverschlüsse erfolgreich wiedereröffnet werden konnten, bei denen die herkömmliche Technik versagte [13]. Perforationen traten nicht auf, histologische und angioskopische Kontrollen des neu entstandenen Kanals zeigten eine relativ glatte Oberfläche. Im folgenden soll über unsere klinischen Erfahrungen bei Patienten mit chronischen Verschlüssen peripherer Arterien berichtet werden.

Material und Methode

Patienten. Im Dezember 1986 begannen wir mit der klinischen Anwendung der Technik [14]; bis Januar 1989 wurden 100 Patienten behandelt. 29 Frauen und 71 Männer im Alter von 35 bis 90 Jahren (mittleres Alter 68,5 Jahre). Bei 62 Patienten war die A. femoralis superficialis, bei 26 Patienten die A. poplitea und bei 12 Patienten die A. iliaca (communis: 8, externa 1, beide Abschnitte 3) chronisch verschlossen. Die Verschlußlängen lagen zwischen 4 und 35 cm mit einer mittleren Verschlußlänge von 12,5 cm. Bei 73 Patienten zeigten die Arterien im Verschlußbereich erhebliche Verkalkungen. Die Patienten wurden in 4 Gruppen unterteilt:

Gruppe 1: 18 Patienten mit Ersteingriff und Verschlüssen der A. femoralis superficialis oder A. poplitea unter 10 cm Länge.
Gruppe 2: 46 Patienten mit Ersteingriff und Verschlüssen der A. femoralis superficialis oder A. poplitea über 10 cm Länge.
Gruppe 3: 24 Patienten nach erfolglosem Versuch der Wiedereröffnung von Verschlüssen der A. femoralis superficialis oder A. poplitea mit herkömmlichen Techniken.
Gruppe 4: 12 Patienten mit chronischen Verschlüssen der A. iliaca; Verschlußlängen zwischen 5 und 20 cm (mittlere Verschlußlänge 9,8 cm).

Klinische und angiographische Vorbefunde

87 Patienten waren im klinischen Stadium IIb, 3 Patienten im Stadium IIa nach Fontaine, die schmerzfreien Gehstrecken lagen zwischen 30 und 300 m (mittlere Gehstrecke 105 m). Bei 10 Patienten bestand ein Stadium IV

mit Nekrosen und Ruheschmerz; 7 von diesen waren als inoperabel von den Gefäßchirurgen eingestuft worden und es drohte die Amputation. Der Bein-/Arm-Doppler-Quotient vor Behandlung lag zwischen 0 und 0,86 (im Mittel bei 0,53).

Nach anamnestischen Angaben (gefragt wurde, wie lange die Klaudikationsbeschwerden in der jetzt vorliegenden Ausprägung bestanden) konnte die Verschlußdauer auf 5–48 Monate geschätzt werden; bei 7 Patienten waren Mindestverschlußzeiten von 6 bis 36 Monaten durch angiographische Voruntersuchungen belegt.

Untersuchungsablauf

Eine flexible Welle von 2,2 mm Außendurchmesser, bestehend aus 4 × 0,2 mm V2A-Stahlschraubendrähten mit Innenlumen zur Einführung eines Wechseldrahtes und Injektion von Kontrastmittel, umhüllt von einem Teflonschrumpfschlauch und mit olivenförmigem, stumpfem Kopf (Abb. 1) wird von einem Elektromotor angetrieben. Dieser Motor ist stufenlos regelbar von 0–500 U/min. Zu Beginn unserer Untersuchungen wurde die Drehgeschwindigkeit bei Netzanschluß über einen Trafo mit Fußschalter geregelt [14], das endgültige Modell wird von einer 9-Volt-Batterie angetrieben, wobei die Umdrehungszahl stufenlos über ein Potentiometer am Gerät gewählt werden kann (Abb. 2).*

Nach antegrader Punktion der A. femoralis communis und Injektion von 5000 Einheiten Heparin intraarteriell wurde eine konventionelle 7- oder 8-French-Schleuse eingelegt und eine angiographische Darstellung der gesamten Extremität durchgeführt. Mit Hilfe der digitalen Subtraktionsangiographie (DSA) wurde dann ein Standbild der Verschlußstrecke angefertigt, das dem Live-Durchleuchtungsbild wie eine Landkarte unterlegt werden konnte (road mapping).

Bei den 12 Patienten mit Verschlüssen der A. iliaca, die erst nach mehr als einjähriger Erfahrung mit der neuen Technik behandelt wurden, erfolgte zunächst eine retrograde Punktion der A. femoralis communis der Gegenseite. Daraufhin wurde mit Hilfe eines 4-F-Pigtailkatheters in der Aorta abdominalis ein Standbild angefertigt und die A. femoralis communis auf der Seite des vorgeschalteten Verschlusses bei unterlegtem road-mapping-Bild retrograd punktiert. Dieses Vorgehen erleichtert sowohl das Auffinden der Arterie bei fehlendem Leistenpuls als auch das vorsichtige Einführen der Schleuse bei relativ kurzem distalen Gefäßstummel.

Der Rotationskatheter wurde direkt durch die Plastikmembrandichtung in die Schleuse eingeführt und unter Durchleuchtungskontrolle bis zum Verschluß vorgeschoben (auf die zu Beginn der klinischen Untersuchungen entwickelten komplizierten Rotationsschleusen (vgl. 14) konnte in der Folge durch technische Änderungen an den Motoren verzichtet werden). Bei Erreichen des Verschlusses wurde der in der rechten Hand des Untersuchers liegende kleine Elektromotor gestartet und die Verschlußstrecke mit Rotationsgeschwindigkeiten von 100–200 U/min und unter geringem axialen Schub unter kontinuierlicher Durchleuchtungskontrolle passiert (Abb. 3). Wenn die Wiederauffüllung distal erreicht schien, wurde

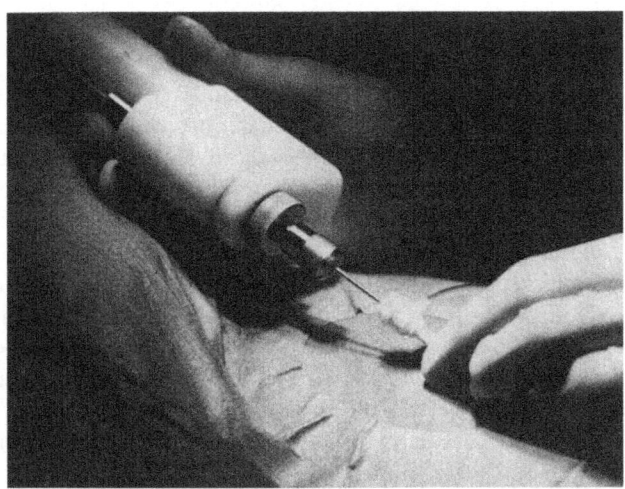

Abb. 3. Die linke Hand des Untersuchers hält die Schleuse, in der rechten Hand liegt der Elektromotor, in den der Rotationskatheter eingespannt ist

nach Aspiration von Blut zunächst Kontrastmittel durch den Rotationskatheter injiziert, um die korrekte Lage im Gefäßlumen zu dokumentieren. Dann wurde der bis zu diesem Zeitpunkt im Rotationskatheter (etwa 2 cm hinter dem Kopf) liegende 0,35"-Wechseldraht nach distal vorgeschoben. Nach Rückzug des Rotationskatheters wurde der neu entstandene Kanal bei liegendem Wechseldraht angiographisch dokumentiert und anschließend mit einem herkömmlichen Ballonkatheter dilatiert.

Medikamentöse Behandlung

Alle Patienten erhielten Acetylsalicylsäure in einer Dosierung von 0,5–1,5 g/die [1], beginnend mindestens 24 Stunden vor dem Eingriff und bis zum Zeitpunkt der angiographischen Kontrolluntersuchung (in der Regel nach etwa 6 Monaten). Während des Eingriffs erfolgte eine kontinuierliche Perfusion der Schleuse mit einer Kombination aus 2000 Einheiten Heparin und 100 000 Einheiten Urokinase pro Stunde; diese Perfusion entspricht unserem Vorgehen bei der Koronarangioplastik, wo systematische Untersuchungen der Führungsdrähte hierunter signifikant weniger Fibrinauflagerungen zeigten [9]. Unmittelbar nach dem Eingriff folgte eine kontrollierte intravenöse Heparingabe von 1000–1200 E/h über 48 Stunden. Nur in Einzelfällen (sehr lange Verschlußstrecken, Unverträglichkeit von Acetylsalicylsäure) wurde eine Dauerantikoagulation durchgeführt. Seit einem halben Jahr verzichten wir auf die erwähnte Perfusion mit 100 000 E Urokinase/h, was zu keinerlei Änderung der Akuterfolgs- oder Komplikationsraten geführt hat.

Ergebnisse

Angiographische Ergebnisse:

Gruppe 1: (18 Patienten mit Ersteingriff und Verschlüssen der A. femoralis superficialis oder A. poplitea unter 10

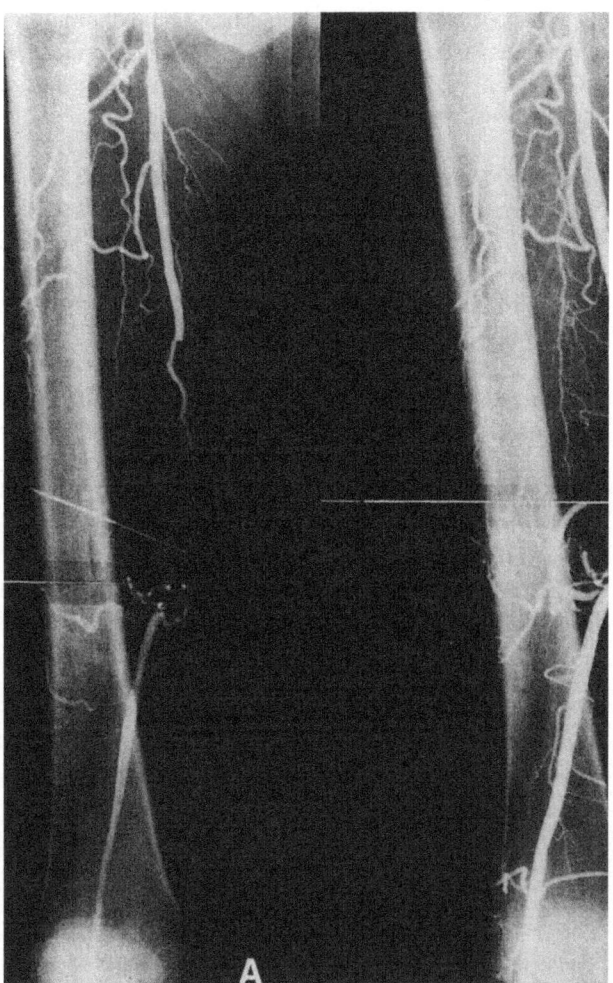

Abb. 4. 11 cm langer chronischer Verschluß der A. femoralis superficialis, der mit herkömmlichen Techniken 4 Wochen zuvor nicht zu eröffnen war. **A)** vor und **B)** nach Rotationsangioplastik und Ballondilatation

cm Länge; im Mittel bei 5,8 cm): Bei 17 von 18 Patienten konnten die Verschlüsse erfolgreich wiedereröffnet werden.

Gruppe 2: (46 Patienten mit Ersteingriff und Verschlüssen der A. femoralis superficialis oder A. poplitea über 10 cm Länge; im Mittel bei 14,8 cm, längster Verschluß 35 cm): Bei 38 von 46 Patienten war die Wiedereröffnung erfolgreich.

Gruppe 3: (24 Patienten nach erfolglosem Versuch der Wiedereröffnung mit herkömmlichen Angioplastietechniken; bei 3 Patienten nach mehr als einem Versuch. Mittlere Verschlußlänge 10,5 cm): 20 von 24 Patienten wurden mit der Rotationsangioplastik mehr als 4 Wochen nach dem erfolglosen konventionellen Versuch behandelt: bei 13 von 20 konnten die Verschlüsse erfolgreich wiedereröffnet werden (Abb. 4). 4 von 24 Patienten wurden weniger als 4 Wochen nach dem erfolglosen konventionellen Versuch behandelt: hier war nur bei einem Patienten eine Rekanalisation zu erreichen.

Gruppe 4: (12 Patienten mit chronischen Verschlüssen der A. iliaca; mittlere Verschlußlänge 9,8 cm): Bei 7 von 12 Patienten konnten die Verschlüsse erfolgreich wiedereröffnet werden. Bei 2 Patienten wurde aufgrund deutlicher Reste von thrombotischem Material im ehemals verschlossenen Bereich eine lokale Lyse mit Urokinase angeschlossen; bei einem Patienten mit einer elastischen Stenose wurde ein 8-mm-stent implantiert.

Gründe für nichterfolgreiche Eingriffe

Gefäße, bei denen sich unter Durchleuchtung "schollenförmige" Verkalkungen im Verschlußbereich zeigten, die z. T. spürbar den gesamten Gefäßquerschnitt verlegten, erwiesen sich als nicht rekanalisierbar. Die teilweise sehr ausgeprägten Verkalkungen der Arterienwand, die den Gefäßverlauf nachzeichnen, beeinträchtigten die Erfolgsaussichten dagegen nicht. In vier Fällen zeigten sich bei sehr langer Verschlußdauer besonders stark ausgeprägte proximale Kollateralgefäße, die ohne wesentlichen Winkel den Verlauf des originären Gefäßes fortsetzten. Da ein eigentlicher proximaler Gefäßstummel fehlte, glitten der Rotationskatheter wie auch die konventionellen Führungsdrähte immer wieder in diese Kollateralen. Eine Verletzung der Kollateralgefäße trat hierdurch nicht auf.

Komplikationen

Perforationen oder andere schwerwiegende Komplikationen durch den Rotationskatheter traten nicht auf. Wir beobachteten 7 folgenlose Dissektionen, eine kleine periphere Embolie ohne klinische Konsequenzen und bei 5 Patienten ein größeres Hämatom an der Punktionsstelle, das bei einem Patienten eine chirurgische Revision und eine Transfusion erforderlich machte.

Funktionelle Ergebnisse

Bei den 75 erfolgreich behandelten Patienten stieg der Bein-/Arm-Doppler-Quotient (gemessen am 2. Tag nach dem Eingriff) von im Mittel 0,53 auf im Mittel 0,89 an. Bei 4 der 7 als inoperabel von den Gefäßchirurgen abgelehnten Patienten im Stadium IV konnte die erfolgreiche Wiederöffnung die drohende Amputation verhindern und ein Stadium IIb erreicht werden. Eine Verschlechterung trat in keinem Fall ein.

Erste angiographisch kontrollierte Langzeitergebnisse

Bis März 1989 konnten 31 Patienten angiographisch nach 2 bis 28 Wochen (im Mittel nach 16,4 Wochen) kontrolliert werden. Dabei zeigte sich bei 15 Patienten ein gutes Langzeitergebnis ohne hämodynamisch wirksame Stenose, 5 Patienten wiesen im ehemals verschlossenen Gefäßabschnitt nun eine wirksame Stenose auf, und bei 11 Patienten war es zu einem Reverschluß gekommen. Die mittlere Länge der ursprünglichen Verschlüsse lag in der Gruppe der Patienten mit Reverschluß oder Restenose deutlich höher (12,9 cm) als bei Patienten mit gutem Langzeitergebnis (9,9 cm). 11 von 16 Patienten mit Reverschluß oder Restenose wurden erneut mit der Rotationsangioplastik bzw. einer konventionellen Ballondilatation behandelt, 2 Patienten wurden konservativ behandelt, und bei 2 Patienten wurde eine Bypass-Operation durchgeführt. Eine Amputation wurde in keinem Fall erforderlich.

Diskussion

Chronischen arteriellen Gefäßverschlüssen liegen wohl in den meisten Fällen Ulzerationen der arteriosklerotischen Plaques zugrunde, die zum Verschluß des letzten Lumens durch sich auflagernde Thromben führten. Dieser pathophysiologische Ablauf bedingt zwei wesentliche Folgerungen; zum einen ist die Gefahr der Dissektion oder gar Wandperforation bei dem Versuch der mechanischen Wiedereröffnung durch die präformierten Einrisse deutlich erhöht und steigt mit zunehmender Verschlußlänge weiter an, zum anderen verbleibt über unterschiedlich lange Zeit im Verschlußquerschnitt eine „weiche Stelle", eben dieser letztlich verschließende Thrombus, der den Weg in das letzte Lumen weist.

Ein relativ dünner und gerader Draht, wie er bisher allgemein zur Rekanalisation verwendet wird, kann sehr leicht in solche vorbestehenden Wandrisse eintreten; selbst bei erfolgreichem Wiedereintritt in das Gefäßlumen entsteht hierdurch ein Neolumen, dessen Akut- und Langzeitergebnisse unbefriedigend sind. Wird solch ein Draht durch eine vorgeschaltete Gefäßbiegung gegen der veränderte Wand gelenkt, so steigt die Gefahr der Wandperforation.

Unsere neue Technik der Rotationsangioplastik [6, 13, 14] verwendet anstelle eines solchen dünnen Drahtes einen relativ weitlumigen, flexiblen und durch die spezielle Kopfform ideal stumpfen Katheter. Die langsame Rotation führt zu einer weitgehenden Aufhebung der Haftreibung, wodurch die Vorwärtsbewegung erleichtert, Gefäßbiegungen leicht verfolgt und Widerstände besonders sensitiv nach proximal übertragen werden.

All diese Eigenschaften bedingen eine deutlich niedrigere Tendenz zur Dissektion; die Gefahr der Wandperforation scheint nach unseren bisherigen experimentellen und klinischen Untersuchungen praktisch nicht gegeben zu sein. Von Hochgeschwindigkeitsrotationstechniken [8, 11] unterscheidet sich unser Verfahren sowohl technisch als auch im Grundkonzept. Während diese mit Drehgeschwindigkeiten bis 150 000 U/min und z. T. diamantbesetzten, scharfen Bohrköpfen eine Abrasion von Verschlußmaterial anstreben, handelt es sich bei der Rotationsangioplastik um eine Verdrängung bzw. Kompression und Volumenreduktion durch Flüssigkeitsabpressung [7]; der Ablauf gleicht einer stumpfen Präparation. Trifft der olivenförmige, stumpfe Kopf unter leichtem axialen Schub auf den Verschlußquerschnitt, so beginnt ein „Suchen" nach dem Weg des geringsten Widerstandes. Da der letztlich verschließende Thrombus in seiner Organisation und Verhärtung den übrigen Verschlußanteilen „nachhinkt", stellt er für lange Zeit (wohl z. T. bis zu mehreren Jahren) den Ort des leichtesten Eindringens dar. Die Passage des Rotationskatheters wird also in aller Regel durch das letzte "wahre" Lumen erfolgen; die sich in jedem Fall anschließende Ballondilatation ergibt wohl aus diesem Grunde oft sehr glatte Konturen.

Unsere experimentellen und jetzt schon über 2 Jahre reichenden klinischen Erfahrungen zeigen, daß die Wiedereröffnung mit dem langsam rotierenden, stumpfen Katheter ein besonders schonendes und sicheres Verfahren

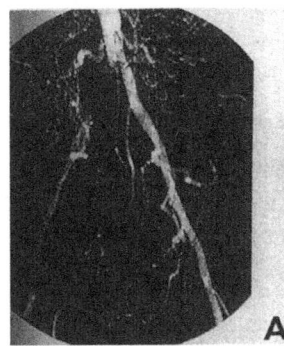 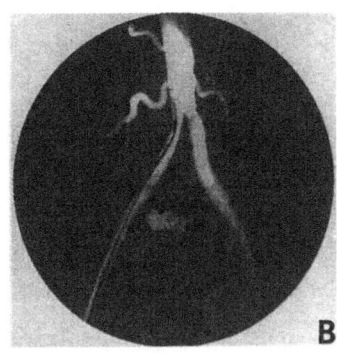

Abb. 5. Chronischer Verschluß der A. iliaca communis rechts. **A)** vor und **B)** nach Rotationsangioplastik und Ballondilatation. (Man erkennt den noch liegenden Wechseldraht)

ist; Perforationen oder andere schwerwiegende Komplikationen traten in keinem Fall auf. Die Akuterfolgsrate bei Ersteingriff liegt über 80 %; auch sehr langstreckige Verschlüsse konnten erfolgreich wiedereröffnet werden. Diese Ergebnisse liegen deutlich über denen herkömmlicher Angioplastietechniken. Bleiben Wiedereröffnungsversuche mit konventionellen Techniken erfolglos, so kann der Rotationskatheter bei einem zeitlichen Mindestabstand von 4 Wochen zum Ersteingriff noch in mehr als 60 % diese bisher nicht behandelbaren Verschlüsse erfolgreich rekanalisieren. Der zeitliche Abstand erscheint erforderlich, um die durch den konventionellen Versuch der Wiedereröffnung entstandenen Dissektionswege verheilen zu lassen.

Neben der Ausweitung der Indikationen auf die A. iliaca (Abb. 5) werden renale und koronare Gefäßverschlüsse in Zukunft mit in die Indikation einbezogen werden können. Die ersten vorliegenden angiographisch dokumentierten Langzeitergebnisse sind ermutigend, bedürfen aber bei noch zu geringer Zahl und zu kurzen Zeiträumen der weiteren sorgfältigen Untersuchung.

Schlußfolgerungen

1. Die neue Technik der Rotationsangioplastik benutzt zur Wiedereröffnung chronisch verschlossener Arterien einen relativ dicken, flexiblen, durch die olivenförmige Kopfform ideal stumpfen, langsam rotierenden Katheter, der von einem kleinen Elektromotor angetrieben wird.
2. Die Rate der erfolgreichen Wiedereröffnung chronisch verschlossener Arterien mit diesem neuen Verfahren liegt deutlich über derjenigen konventioneller Techniken.
3. Bisher nicht behandelbare Verschlüsse können noch in mehr als 60 % der Fälle erfolgreich wiedereröffnet werden.
4. Das neue Verfahren ist besonders schonend: Perforationen oder andere schwerwiegende Komplikationen traten in keinem Fall auf.

Literatur

1. Breddin HK: Treatment with platelet function inhibitors. In: Kaltenbach M, Grüntzig A, Rentrop K, Bussmann WD (eds.): Transluminal coronary angioplasty and intracoronary thrombolysis. Springer, Heidelberg (1982) 41–43
2. Dotter DC, Judkins MP: Transluminal treatment of arteriosclerotic obstruction: Description of a new technique and a preliminary report of its application. Circulation 30 (1964) 654
3. Faxon DP, Kelsey S, Kellet MA, Ryan TJ, Detre K: And members of the NHLBI PTCA-Registry: Predictors of a successful angioplasty (PTCA-registry). Circulation 74 (1986) 768
4. Graziani L: Percutaneous recanalization of total iliac and femoro-popliteal artery occlusions. Eur J Radiol 7 (1987) 91–93
5. Grüntzig A, Hopff H: Perkutane Rekanalisation chronischer arterieller Verschlüsse mit einem neuen Dilatationskatheter. Modifikation der Dottertechnik. Dtsch Med Wschr 99 (1974) 2502–2510
6. Kaltenbach M, Vallbracht C: Rotationsangioplastik – ein neues Katheterverfahren. Fortschr Med 105 (1987) 412–414
7. Kaltenbach M, Beyer J, Klepzig H, Schmidts L, Hübner K: Effect of 5 kg/cm² pressure on atherosclerotic wall segments. In: Kaltenbach M, Grüntzig A, Rentrop K, Bussmann WD (eds.): Transluminal coronary angioplasty and intracoronary thrombolysis. Springer, Heidelberg (1982) 189–193
8. Kensey RK, Nash JE, Abrahams C, Zarius CHK: Recanalization of obstructed arteries with a flexible, rotating tip catheter. Radiology 165 (1987) 387–389
9. Kober G, Vallbracht C, Lang H, Bussmann WD, Hopf R, Kunkel B, Kaltenbach M: Transluminale koronare Angioplastik 1977–1985: Erfahrungen bei 1000 Eingriffen. Radiologe 25 (1985) 346
10. Mathias K, Gospos CH, Thron A et al.: Percutaneous transluminal treatment of supraaortic artery obstructions. Ann Radiol 23 (1980) 281
11. Ritchie JL, Hansen DD, Vracko H, Auth D: In vivo rotational thrombectomy-evaluation by angiocopy. Circulation, Vol. 74, Suppl II: 1822 (1986) (abstr.)
12. Simpson JB, Blaim DS, Robert E, Harrison DC: A new catheter system for coronary angioplasty. Amer J Cardiol 49 (1982) 1216–1222
13. Vallbracht C, Kress J, Schweitzer M, Schneider M, Wendt Th, Ziemen M, Kollath J, Bamberg W, Kaltenbach M: Rotationsangioplastik – ein neues Verfahren zur Gefäßwiedereröffnung und -erweiterung. Experimentelle Befunde. Z Kardiol 76 (1987) 608–611
14. Vallbracht C, Schweitzer M, Kress J, Bamberg W, Kollath J, Liermann D, Paasch C, Rauber K, Roth FJ, Prignitz I, Beinborn W, Landgraf H, Breddin HK, Schoop W, Kaltenbach M: Rotationsangioplastik – erste klinische Ergebnisse bei peripheren Gefäßverschlüssen. Z Kardiol 77 (1988) 352–357
15. Zeitler E: Die perkutane transluminale Rekanalisation chronischer Stenosen und Verschlüsse peripherer Arterien. Wien. Med Wschr 135 (1985) 384–392

Reopening of Chronic Coronary Artery Occlusions by Low Speed Rotational Angioplasty

M. KALTENBACH and C. VALLBRACHT

Following successful application in chronic peripheral artery occlusions, rotational angioplasty was refined and miniaturized for application in patients with chronic coronary artery occlusions. The new catheter system comprises a motor-driven rotating inner steel catheter made up of several steel coils providing maximum elasticity and complete torque control with an olive-like rounded tip (1.0–1.7 mm). The catheter has a lumen for contrast injection and a shielding plastic tube. It is introduced through a conventional 8 Fr guiding catheter. The slowly rotating (200 RPM) catheter passes nontraumatically through the occlusions, thus creating a new channel with smooth contours in a "remodeling" fashion. Once the channel (diameter 1–1.5 mm) is confirmed angiographically, balloon angioplasty is performed over an exchange wire in conventional technique. The new technique was applied to patients with chronic coronary occlusions. Reopening was first attempted with conventional guide wire technique. If the occlusion could be probed with the guidewire, patients were excluded from the study. Twenty patients in whom the occlusion could not be probed with a wire were studied: 1 ACVB, 2 LAD, and 17 RCA. Average duration of occlusion was 7.4 months; it exceeded 3 months in 15/20 and 6 months in 12/20 patients. Successful reopening was achieved in 9/20 (3 from the first 10, 6 from the second 10 patients). No vessel wall perforation or any other severe complication was encountered. Residual stenosis diameter ranged from 30%–70%. Duration of occlusion was similar among patients from the successful and unsuccessful group. It is concluded that with low speed rotational angioplasty reopening of chronic coronary artery occlusions can be achieved in a considerable part of patients in whom conventional technique is unsuccessful. (J Interven Cardiol 1989:2:3)

Introduction

Techniques for reopening chronic arterial occlusions must be separated into those designed to pass the occlusion for the first time and those applied via a wire with which the lesion has been previously passed.

It is evident that once a wire has been advanced beyond the occluded part of the vessel, one can introduce different tools without danger since the wire provides safe guidance. Hot-tip catheters [1], laser catheters [2], and endarterectomy catheters [3–5] have been applied instead of, or in addition to, conventional balloon catheters.

The main problem remains the primary passage of a totally occluded artery. With presently available techniques, the passage of fresh and subacute occlusions is possible in the majority of patients, the success rate, however, drops steeply with duration of occlusion and "is almost zero in obstructions older than 6 months" [6]. New techniques such as laser or hot-tip devices have been attempted over many years. Their application appears, however, to be limited mainly due to the risk of vessel wall perforation.

Rotational angioplasty is a new technique designed to circumvent these difficulties [7]. It has proven to allow reopening of chronic peripheral artery occlusions with a high success rate and no danger of vessel wall perforation [8–11]. The method was refined and miniaturized for application in chronic coronary artery occlusions. The results obtained in the first 20 patients will be reported in this paper.

Method

The rotational angioplasty catheter system is introduced through a conventional 8 Fr guiding catheter. It comprises an inner steel catheter and a shielding plastic catheter. The shielding catheter consists of a polyethylene or polyolefine tube with a contrast marker at its distal end. The rotating inner catheter has a shaft made from several stainless steel coils. The small diameter of the stainless steel wire material and the combination of several coils provides maximal elasticity combined with complete torque control. The tip of the steel catheter consists of an olive-like rounded tip with a diameter ranging from 1.0 to 1.7 mm. Rotation is achieved by a sterile battery-driven electric motor with a low speed of roughly 200 RPM (Fig. 1).

Patients

In patients with chronic coronary artery occlusions treated from April 1987 until February 1988, the occlusion was first probed with conventional guidewires. If the wire passed the occlusion, patients were excluded from the study. Twenty patients (1 female, 19 male) in whom the occlusion could not be passed with a wire were included in the study. One had an occluded aorto-coronary LAD venous bypass, 2 an occluded LAD and 17 an occluded RCA. Duration of occlusion estimated from a previous angiogram, from sudden appearance of anginal symptoms or from the occurrence of a myocardial infarction ranged from 1 month to 12 years with an average of 8 months. In

Reprint from J. of Interventional Cardiology Vol. 2, 137–145, 1989, No. 3
Futura Pub., Mount Kisco

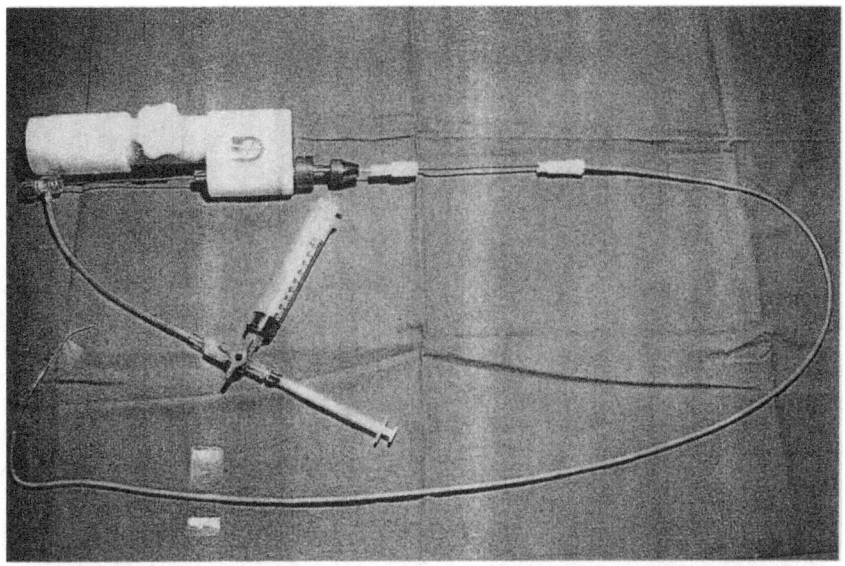

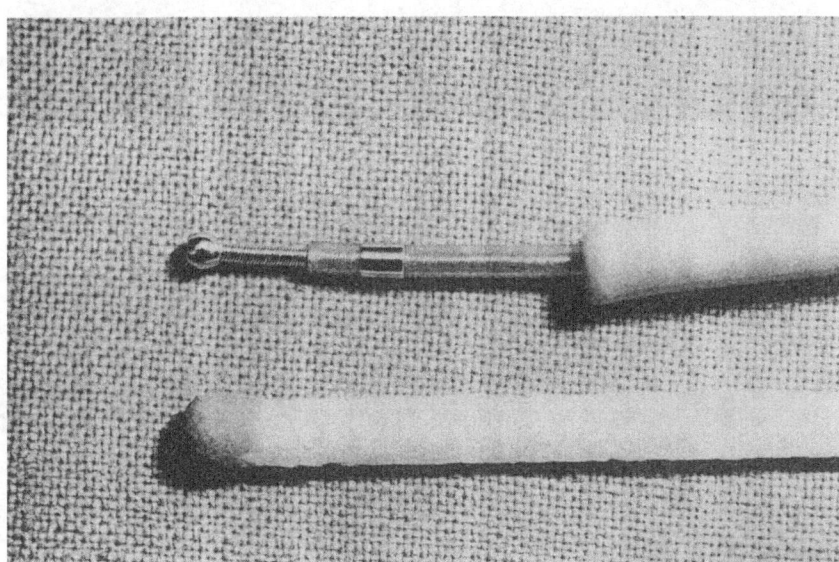

Fig. 1. Low speed rotational angioplasty catheter system: ROTACS (Oscor Medical Corp., Palm Harbor, FL, USA)

75% of cases, it amounted to more than 3 months and in 60% to more than 6 months. All patients had subjective symptoms consisting of exertional angina and/or dyspnea. Exercise testing was performed, before the procedure and 24 hours after reopening the occluded artery. Most patients had a history of myocardial infarction. Left ventricular contraction was at least partially preserved in the postobstructional myocardium.

Procedure

The right or left brachial artery was exposed, coronary angiography performed and the presence of a total occlusion reconfirmed after injecting nitroglycerin intracoronarily. A guiding catheter (8 Fr) was placed into the respective coronary or bypass ostium. The occlusion was probed with a guidewire.

If it was possible to pass the occlusion using a wire, rotational angioplasty was not performed. The patient was

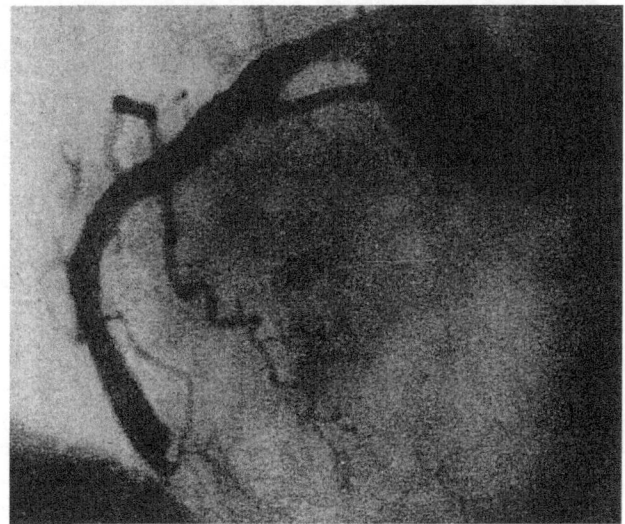

Fig. 2a. Chronic obstruction of a dominant right coronary artery

M. Kaltenbach and L. Vallbracht

Reprint from J. of Interventional Cardiology Vol. 2, 137–145, 1989, No. 3
Futura Pub., Mount Kisco

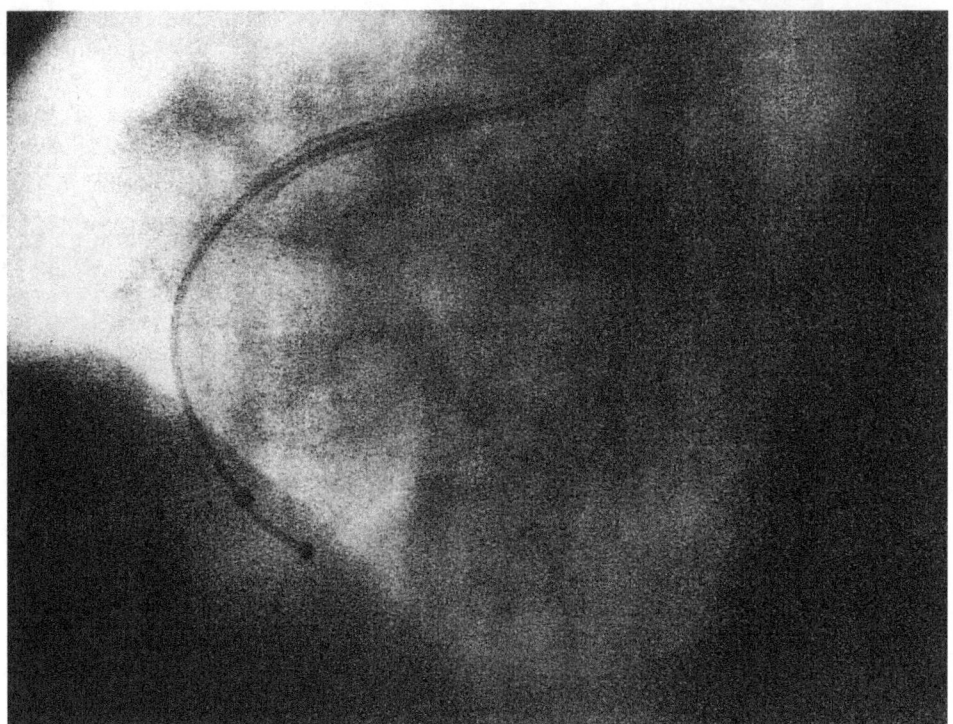

Fig. 2b. Rotational angioplasty catheter passing the obstruction

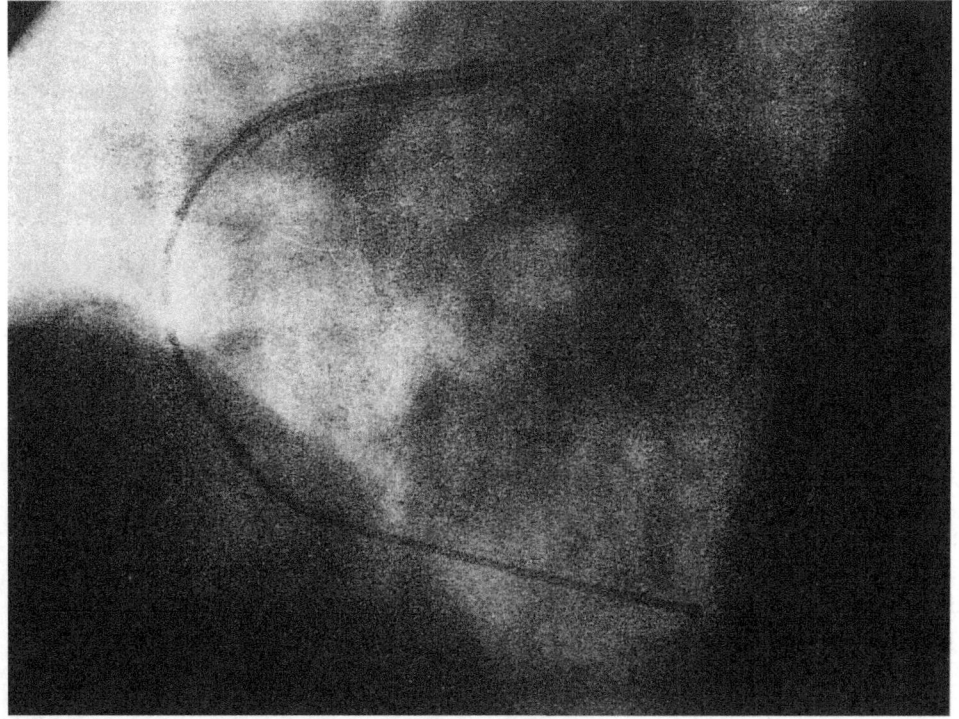

Fig. 2c. Tip of the rotational catheter in the distal artery

then excluded from the study and only conventional balloon angioplasty was performed. In two patients another attempt of reopening the occlusion had been performed without success in a separate previous procedure. The rotational angioplasty catheter system was introduced through a 8 Fr guiding catheter and advanced as far as to the proximal part of the obstruction. The stainless steel inner catheter was then rotated and passage attempted. During this attempt and once the tip of the catheter had

reached the distal coronary artery, contrast material was injected through the free lumen of the rotational catheter. If correct placement in the distal coronary artery was confirmed, an exchange wire was introduced and the rotational catheter removed. By contrast injection through the guiding catheter, the antegrade flow to the distal part of the obstructed artery was confirmed and the channel created by the rotating catheter visualized. A balloon catheter was then introduced over the wire and the chan-

Reprint from J. of Interventional Cardiology Vol. 2, 137–145, 1989, No. 3
Futura Pub., Mount Kisco

nel further dilated (Fig. 2). If necessary, repeat dilatation was performed using a larger balloon.

Antithrombotic measures included acetyl salicylic acid 1.5 g/day, commencing at least 24 hours prior to the procedure. Two-hundred U/kg body weight of heparin were given intra-arterially at the beginning of the procedure. Throughout the procedure, perfusion of the guiding catheter was performed with heparin 2,000 U/h plus urokinase 100,000 U/h. In one case, in which large thrombotic masses were evident in the occluded artery, additional 1.5 million U of urokinase were administered intravenously after the procedure.

Results

In three patients out of the first ten, the occlusion could be passed using the rotating catheter. Of the second ten patients, six attempts proved successful. The successfully treated patient group comprised one patient with an aortocoronary LAD venous bypass, one with a LAD occlusion and seven with RCA occlusions.

The duration of occlusion in this group ranged from 1–12 months ($\overline{X} = 7.4$) and in the unsuccessfully treated patients from 1–124 months ($\overline{X} = 40$). It exceeded 6 months in 60% of patients from each group.

The channel created by the rotational catheter showed a diameter of 1–1.5 mm and always smooth contours in the arteriogram. Its diameter was not considered large enough and therefore further dilated in all patients. The final residual stenosis was 50% in the mean and varied from 30%–70%.

There was no difference between the two patient groups in regard to sex, patient age, obstruction localization or any other clinical or anatomical parameter.

In seven of the nine successfully treated patients, exercise tests were performed before and after the procedure. At the same workload and exercise duration three showed an improvement with regard to angina pectoris and ST-depression, four remained unchanged and none showed any deterioration. Another patient had no exercise test prior to the procedure due to unstable angina. After the procedure his exercise test was normal (Table 1).

Complications

No severe complications (myocardial infarction, emergency operation) were encountered. In one patient thrombotic material from the area of occlusion was displaced by the balloon catheter into the distal vessel without hemodynamic consequences. This displacement did not occur in connection with the reopening by the rotational catheter, it appeared only after expansion of the balloon and had no clinical consequences. In three patients contrast material in the vessel wall indicated vessel wall dissection. There were no hemodynamic consequences. Vessel wall perforation did not occur.

Discussion

Chronic occlusions are the main limitation today for performing nonsurgical revascularization in patients with coronary artery disease. Following favorable experimental results [7, 8], low speed rotational angioplasty was applied to chronically occluded peripheral arteries [9, 10]. When occlusions were extended over a length not exceeding 10 cm, a 95% success rate was achieved. Even in occlusions extended over more than 10 cm, the success rate

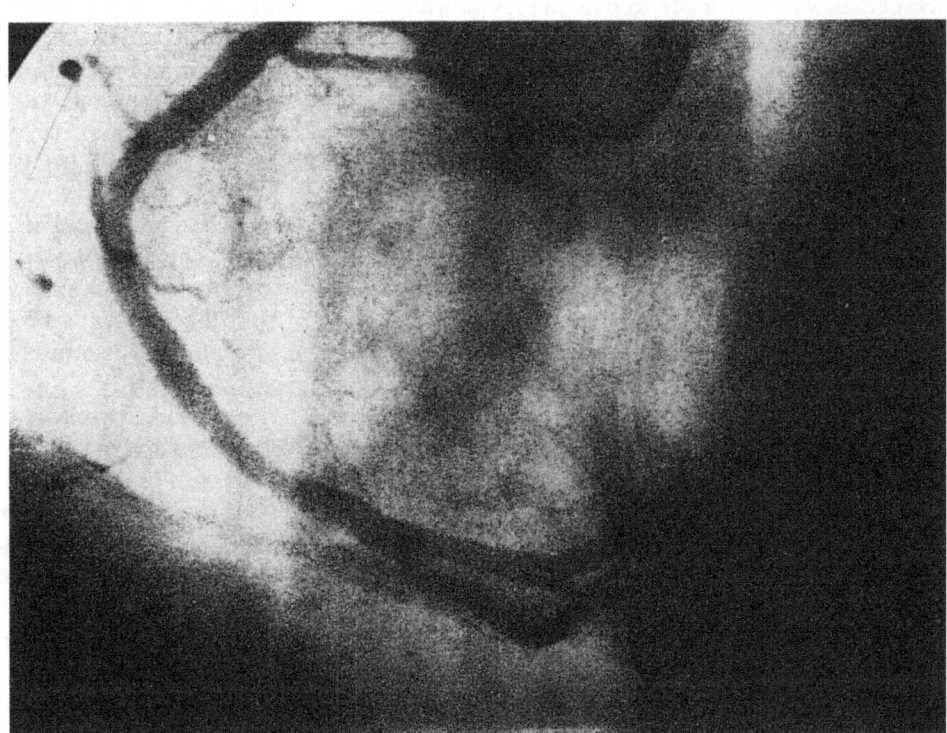

Fig. 2d. Following removal of the rotational catheter, the antegrade flow to the distal vessel and the exchange wire are visible as well as the channel created by the rotational catheter

M. Kaltenbach and L. Vallbracht

Reprint from J. of Interventional Cardiology Vol. 2, 137–145, 1989, No. 3
Futura Pub., Mount Kisco

30

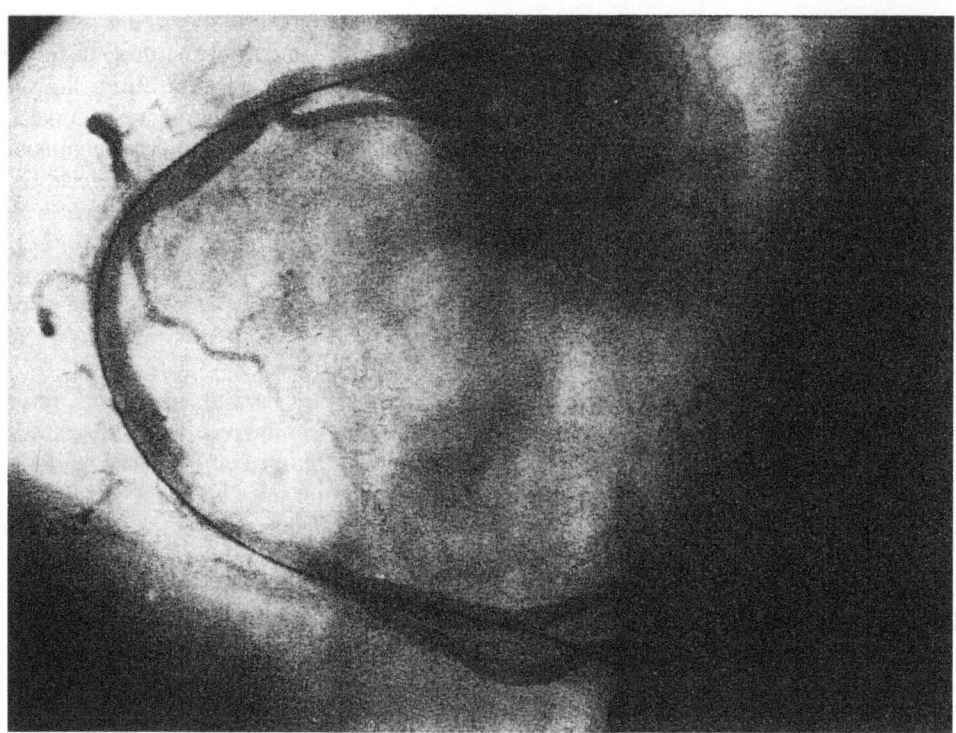

Fig. 2e. Good widening of the occluded vessel segment after balloon angioplasty

amounted to 75 %. In cases where one or several previous attempts with conventional techniques had failed, the success rate was still 65 %. Most importantly, there has not been any vessel wall perforation in more than 80 patients [10].

After miniaturizing and refining the catheter system, the method was applied to 20 patients with chronic coronary artery occlusions. In the majority of patients, occlusion duration exceeded 6 months. It is known that the success rate with conventional technique is low under these circumstances [5, 6]. In the present study, an attempt with each patient was first made to pass the lesion using conventional guidewires. Rotational angioplasty was only attempted in patients in whom the obstruction could not be passed with a guidewire. In two patients, the attempt of reopening the vessel with conventional techniques had failed in a previous intervention 1 and 11 months, respectively, earlier, in the other patients the first attempt was made in the same session before applying rotational angioplasty.

The essential characteristic of the new catheter system is its excellent torque control combined with high flexibility. The rounded tip with a relatively large diameter further minimizes the danger of vessel wall penetration. The catheter is not intended to penetrate hard obstructions, but to find a way through the softest part of the obstructing tissue, i.e., usually the nonorganized remainders of the occlusive thrombus.

The rotating catheter is neither designed nor has any properties to displace atherosclerotic or thrombotic material. The channel within the obstruction is created by pressing fluid or soft material outward [12]. This process of remodeling is similar to the mechanism of balloon angioplasty and the term "rotational angioplasty" was, thus, considered appropriate.

The ability of the slowly rotating catheter to advance in a nontraumatic fashion is attributed to the high flexibility of the catheter shaft and the olive-shaped thickened distal tip. Rotation at a low speed of 200 RPM is sufficient to reduce friction and allow sensitive longitudinal movement of the catheter tip.

Experience gained from 20 patients indicates that this new method of revascularization may be used in cases where otherwise only surgery was possible. The patient population comprised predominantly RCA occlusions. This was to some part the consequence of respective transferrals and to another of the intention to begin with a group of patients at lowest risk.

From earlier experience obtained in patients with chronic coronary occlusions with conventional techniques, in our hands, RCA and LAD obstructions had a similar success rate of about 40 % [6]. If one considers that in the present study all patients were excluded in whom conventional technique was successful, the overall success rate using both techniques may be estimated to be 70 %. From 100 patients 40 may respond to conventional techniques and from the remaining 60 patients 30 (50 %) to rotational angioplasty. This would correspond to a total success rate of 70 %.

The typical indication for reopening chronic coronary occlusions are patients in whom the postocclusional myocardium is preserved and responsible for ischemic symptoms. Another indication may exist in patients in whom angioplasty of one vessel with a high grade stenosis cannot be performed because another collateral-providing vessel is totally occluded.

The favorable results obtained from the first 20 patients was confirmed in a total of 75 patients treated with the new technique through July 1989. Thus, reference to the additional 55 patients is as yet anecdotal. Complication

Table 1. Data of the 20 patients submitted to rotational coronary angioplasty. Acute result: 0 = no reopening achieved. Numbers indicate the achieved diameter reduction. Exercise-ECG: Results before and after rotational angioplasty

Patient	Sex	Age	Occluded Artery	Estimated Duration of Occlusion	Acute Result	Complication	Exercise-ECG Before	After
1 S.R.	m.	54	RCA	?	0	0		
2 B.B.	m.	39	RCA	?	0	0		
3 S.H.	m.	56	LAD-Bypass	3 weeks	+ (100 → 50%)	0	unstable	75 watts, 6 min no Ap, no IR
4 H.F.	m.	59	RCA	3 months	0	0		
5 S.W.	m.	56	LAD	?	+ (100 → 50%)	0	100 watts, 6 min. Ap(+), IR(+)	100 watts, 6 min. no Ap, IR(+)
6 M.M.	m.	50	RCA	3 years	0	0		
7 N.W.	m.	62	RCA	4 years	0	0		
8 R.K.	m.	65	RCA	?	0	0		
9 H.W.	m.	33	RCA	?	+ (100 → 40%)	0	150 watts, 5 min. Ap(+), IR(+)	150 watts, 6 min. no Ap, no IR
10 M.H.	m.	74	RCA	posterior infarction 1975	0	0		
11 N.F.	m.	56	RCA	posterior infarction 1979	0	0		
12 P.L.	m.	40	RCA	4 weeks	0	0		
13 M.G.	f.	56	RCA	5 months	+ (100 → 30%)	0	125 watts, 6 min. no Ap, no IR	125 watts, 6 min. no Ap, no IR
14 J.J.	m.	36	LAD	9 months	+ (100 → 70%)	dissection	100 watts, 2 min. Ap(++), IR(+)	
15 S.W.	m.	45	RCA	?	+ (100 → 50%)	0	200 watts, 6 min. no Ap, IR(+)	225 watts, 4 min. no Ap, IR(+)
16 M.J.	m.	57	RCA	4 weeks	0	dissection		
17 G.G.	m.	52	RCA	?	+ (100 → 50%)	0	150 watts, 6 min. no Ap, IR(+)	150 watts, 4 min. no Ap, IR(+)
18 S.K.	m.	58	RCA	1 year	+ (100 → 50%)	peripheral embolism	125 watts, 5 min. Ap(+), IR(+)	125 watts, 3 min. Ap(+), IR(+)
19 G.D.	m.	50	RCA	10 months	+ (100 → 50%)	0	150 watts, 6 min. Ap(++), no IR	150 watts, 6 min. Ap(+), no IR
20 B.O.	m.	50	RCA	11 months	0	dissection		

rate remained low in this larger group including more patients with chronic LAD obstructions. No vessel wall perforation occurred. In several other patients the technique was applied if after successful probing of a high grade stenosis the balloon catheter could not be advanced over the guidewire. In this situation, the low speed rotational catheter was applied over the guidewire and by low rotation a channel could be created allowing the introduction of the balloon catheter.

It is concluded that rotational angioplasty has the potential to allow nonsurgical revascularization in a considerable part of patients with total chronic coronary artery obstructions not responding to conventional techniques.

Acknowledgment: We thank Prof. Satter and his team for surgical standby.

References

1. Cumberland DC, Tayler DI, Welsh CL, et al. Percutaneous laser thermal angioplasty: Initial clinical results with a laser probe in total peripheral artery occlusions. Lancet 1986; 1: 1457–1459

2. Geschwind R, Boussignac G, Teisseire B, et al. Conditions for effective Nd-Yag laser angioplasty. Br Heart J 1984; 52: 484–489

3. Hansen DD, Hall M, Intlekofer MJ, et al. In vivo rotational angioplasty in atherosclerotic rabbits; comparison of angioscopy and angiography (abstr) Circulation 1986; 74 (Suppl. II): II–1443

4. Kensey K, Nash J, Abrahams C, et al. Recanalization of obstructed arteries using a flexible rotating tip catheter. (abstr) Circulation 1986; 74 (Suppl. II): II–457

5. Meier B. Coronary Angioplasty. Orlando, Florida, Grune & Stratton Inc., 1987

6. Kober G, Hopf R, Reinemer H, et al. Langzeitergebnisse der transluminalen koronaren Angioplastie von chronischen Herzkranzgefäßverschlüssen. Z Kardiol 1985; 74: 309–316

7. Kaltenbach M, Vallbracht C. Rotationsangioplastik – ein neues Katheterverfahren für die nicht-operative Gefäßeröffnung. Fortschr Med 1987; 112: 842–844

8. Simpson JB, Johnson DE, Thapliyal HV, et al. Transluminal atherectomy: A new approach to the treatment of atherosclerotic vascular disease. (abstr) Circulation 1985: 72 (Suppl. III): III–146

9. Vallbracht C, Kress J, Schweitzer M, et al. Rotationsangioplastik – ein neues Verfahren zur Gefäßwiedereröffnung und -erweiterung. Z Kardiol 1987; 76: 608–611

10. Vallbracht C, Liermann D, Roth FJ, et al. Results of lowspeed rotational angioplasty for chronic peripheral occlusions. Am J Cardiol 1988; 62: 935–940

11. Vallbracht C, Dieter D, Liermann D, et al. Low-speed rotational angioplasty in chronic femoral and popliteal occlusions: Experiences in 52 patients. Radiology 1988; 169 (Suppl): 387–1289

12. Kaltenbach M, Beyer J, Walter S, et al. Prolonged application of pressure in transluminal coronary angioplasty. Cath Cardiovasc Diag 1984; 10: 213–219

Abstracts

Low Speed Rotational Angioplasty in Chronic Coronary Artery Obstructions

M. KALTENBACH and C. VALLBRACHT

Between 2/87 and 4/89 low speed rotational angioplasty (RA) was attempted in 60 patients (p). RA was performed with a very flexible stainless steel catheter rotated by an electric motor at a low speed of 200 rpm. After passing the obstruction, further widening was achieved by balloon angioplasty. A total of 60 occlusions (RCA = 46, LAD = 8, CX = 4, ACVB = 2) were attempted. The duration of occlusion estimated from previous myocardial infarction, sudden onset of symptoms or previous angiograms was 1 month (m) to 15 years, mean: 8.2 m. Re-opening with conventional guide wires was always tried prior to RA. If the wire passed the occlusion, p were excluded from the study except for 2, in whom the balloon could not be passed over the wire. In these 2 p, RA was performed over the long wire in place; only after a channel had been created by RA, could the balloon be introduced. In this preselected group of p, success rate was about 60%. Complications comprised 1 emergency surgery due to a dissection of the proximal left coronary artery and subsequent narrowing of the CX during an attempt to re-open the occluded LAD. In 1 p thrombotic material from the RCA was embolized distally without clinical consequences. It is concluded that in chronic coronary artery obstructions which cannot be re-opened by conventional techniques, RA is successful in about 60% and has a low complication rate.

Reprint from Circulation Vol. 80 No. 4 Suppl. II, Abstr. 1088

Medium-term Results After Reopening Chronic Coronary Artery Obstructions by Low Speed Rotational Angioplasty

M. KALTENBACH and C. VALLBRACHT

Low speed rotational angioplasty (RA) was performed in 60 patients (p) with chronic coronary obstructions which could not be reopened by conventional techniques. Until April 1989 18 p with successful procedures were followed for at least 4 months. Since recurrences cannot be adequately determined from clinical symptoms and non-invasive studies, follow-up angiography (FA) was proposed to all p.

A total of 17 (95%) of the 18 consecutive p with successful procedures had FA at an average of 3.7 months after the procedure. Three p showed a good result, 8 had restenoses. All 8 p were successfully redilated, 4/8 had a second FA with no further restenosis. Six (35%) of the 17 p had reocclusions.

It is concluded that in p with chronic coronary artery occlusions not responding to conventional techniques but to RA, favourable medium-term results were achieved in 11/17 p (65%).

Low Speed Rotational Angioplasty in Chronic Peripheral Occlusions – First Long-term Results

C. VALLBRACHT, F. J. ROTH, D. LIERMANN, H. LANDGRAF, J. KOLLATH, W. SCHOOP and M. KALTENBACH

Acute and long-term results of conventional angioplasty (PTA) in chronic peripheral occlusions (CPO) have been generally disappointing (acute success rate 50–70%; reocclusion rate up to 60%). Low speed rotational angioplasty (RA) has proven to be a safe and successful techniques even in patients, in whom conventional techniques had failed.

After successful re-opening by RA, 31 p with CPO extended over 5–25 cm (mean 11.5 cm) had an angiographic follow-up study at 2–30 weeks (mean 16.4 weeks). 15/31 p (48%) showed a good long-term result without a significant narrowing, 5/31 p (16%) restenosis (rest) and 11/31 p (36%) reocclusions (reoc). Length of occlusion was higher in p with reoc or rest (mean 12.9 cm) as compared to p with longterm patency (9.9 cm). 11/16 p with reoc or rest underwent a second intervention, two were treated conservatively and in two p bypass surgery was performed. No amputation became necessary.

It is concluded that low speed rotational angioplasty appears a promising procedure in regard to acute and long-term results in patients with chronic peripheral artery occlusions.

Reprint from Circulation Vol. 80 No. 4 Suppl. II, Abstr. 1226

Coronary Balloon Angioplasty

Long Wire Technique – Experience with 1000 Procedures

M. Kaltenbach, C. Vallbracht and G. Kober

Zusammenfassung: Die Langdrahttechnik hat sich bei mehr als 1000 Eingriffen als eine Methode erwiesen, die die Koronarangioplastik leichter und sicherer durchführen läßt. Da die Stenose zunächst nur mit dem Führungsdraht sondiert wird, ist 1. die Kontrastdarstellung während der kritischen Phase der Stenosenpassage unbehindert und 2. sind auch sehr geringe Widerstände beim Vorschieben des Drahtes unmittelbar spürbar. 3. können ohne erneute Sondierung und Traumatisierung Ballonkatheter ausgetauscht werden; im Gegensatz zu verlängerbaren Austauschdrähten sind dabei auch "super-low profile"-Ballonkatheter zu verwenden. 4. Bei Verschluß des Gefäßes kann über den liegenden Führungsdraht das richtige Lumen problemlos sowohl erneut mit einem Ballon als auch mit einem Perfusionskatheter sondiert werden. Die intrakoronare Perfusion mit Eigenblut kann im Bedarfsfall mittels eines einfachen Verbindungssystems als Überbrückung bis zur Bypassoperation durchgeführt werden. 60–100 ml Blut/min können von Hand perfundiert werden. 5. Die Möglichkeit zur intrakoronaren Druckregistrierung bleibt im Gegensatz zum Monorail-System erhalten.

Summary: As shown in more than 1000 procedures the long wire technique has proven its capacity to facilitate coronary angioplasty. Maneuvering of the wire is unhindered because the wire is introduced without a balloon catheter. Optimal contrast display is possible during crossing of the stenosis. Precision and safety of the procedure is therefore considerably improved.
Balloon catheters can be exchanged without recrossing the stenosis including super low profile catheters of small diameter. In case of acute coronary occlusion occurring during angioplasty the long wire allows reintroduction of catheters without danger of via falsa. If necessary a 4.5 F perfusion catheter can be introduced and coronary perfusion with 60–100 ml per minute blood from the femoral artery can be performed by hand. In contrast to the monorail technique the ability to measure pressures through the balloon catheter including intracoronary gradients and coronary capillary pressure is preserved.
Since its introduction in 1977 by Andreas Grüntzig [1] the technique of balloon dilatation has been steadily improved. Today, balloon material is available which can withstand pressures up to 15 kg/cm². The introduction of steerable systems by Simpson has remarkably facilitated the application of angioplasty [2].
Further technical improvements are needed since the method still has a considerable complication rate of the order of up to 1% [3, 4]. The long wire technique is a new approach which further facilitates the procedure and may reduce the complication rate [5, 6].

Key words: coronary angioplasty : long wire technique

---

* 3 m wire 0.012″; Schneider-Medintag, Zürich, Switzerland

Method

Using the long wire technique, the arterial stenosis is first crossed with a special wire of 3 m length*. In contrast to conventional techniques, this wire is introduced without a balloon catheter (Figs. 1 and 2).
During manipulation, the proximal part of the long wire is kept within a tube; therefore the 3 m length of the wire does not hinder the procedure in any way. The rotational and longitudinal movements of the wire are performed with the help of a plastic torquer which is clipped sideways onto the wire and removed from it without pulling the wire out of the tube.
Since fibrin coating and platelet adhesion to the wire may be a possible danger, antithrombotic measures are considered important. We administer acetyl salicylic acid orally (1.5 g/day) beginning at least 1 day before the procedure. At the time of angioplasty the patient receives heparin in a bolus of 100 U/kg body weight. In addition a continuous intraarterial perfusion with heparin 2000 U/h and urokinase 100000 U/h is performed through the guiding catheter. By using teflon-coated wires, the amount of fibrin deposits and platelet adhesion has been considerably reduced. The above perfusion, however, has shown to be of additional efficacy. It is therefore recommended in all procedures.
After having crossed the stenotic area, the tip of the wire is advanced far into the distal coronary artery. In this position another angiogram is performed and displayed as a frozen picture. With this image, an association is achieved between the wire shape and the localization of the stenosis. Thus, accurate positioning of the balloon at the site of the stenosis is facilitated. The proximal part of the wire is taken out of the tube and the appropriate balloon catheter introduced. The balloon catheter is advanced into the stenosis and expanded in the usual way, with continuous pressure monitoring from the guiding catheter and the balloon catheter. If the chosen balloon catheter does not cross a very tight stenosis a smaller

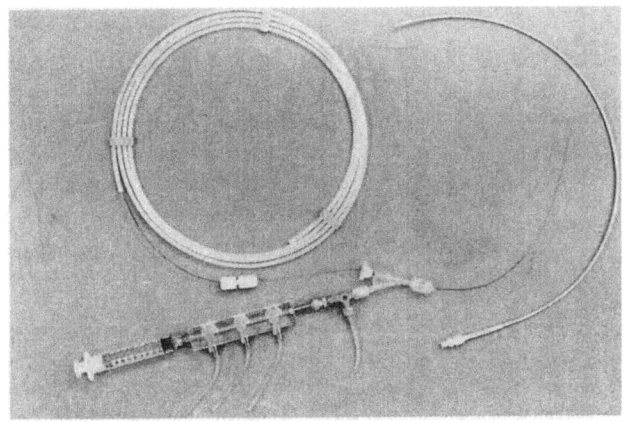

Fig. 1. Equipment for the long wire technique (see text)

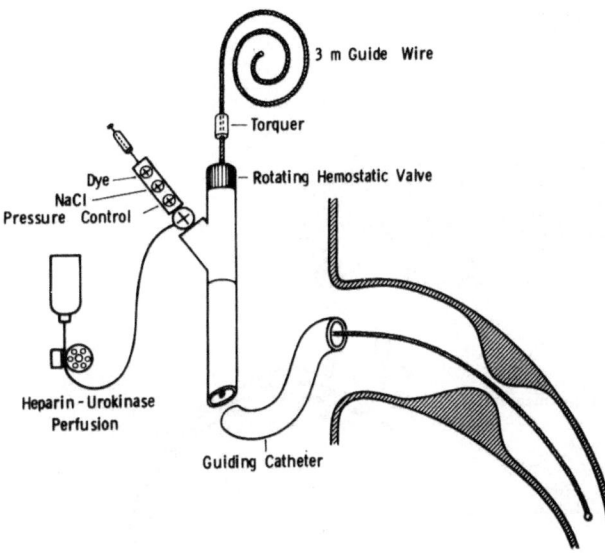

Fig. 2. Principle of the long wire technique: the stenosis is crossed with the wire alone; thereafter, the torquer is removed from the wire and the balloon catheter introduced

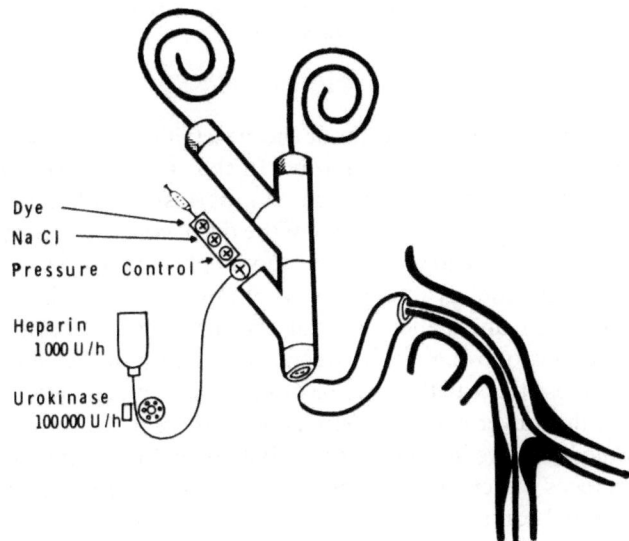

Fig. 3. Application of the long wire technique to branching stenoses. The stenosis is crossed by two long wires introduced through same guiding catheter. Balloon expansion is sequentially performed

balloon catheter, including 2.0 super low profile catheters, can be introduced without difficulty.

After dilatation the balloon catheter is pulled back while the long wire remains within the coronary artery. Then a follow-up angiogram is performed. If the result is not satisfactory, the dilatation can be repeated because the wire remaining in place allows reintroduction of the balloon without risk. Another dilatation can be performed using the same balloon catheter or, if necessary, a balloon catheter with a larger diameter. Only after the control angiogram has shown a satisfactory result is the wire withdrawn.

In the case of branching stenoses, e.g. a stenosis involving the left anterior descending artery and a large diagonal branch, two long wires can be introduced through the same guiding catheter with this technique, one placed in the LAD and one in the diagonal branch. The balloon catheter is then introduced, firstly into the more important vessel. Afterwards, it can be advanced over the second wire to the other branch (Fig. 3). Balloon expansion is performed sequentially.

If acute coronary occlusion occurs during angioplasty, the long wire allows recrossing of the occluded area without risk. Redilatation can be attempted with the same or a larger balloon catheter. If this is unsuccessful, a 4.5 F coronary perfusion catheter can be introduced and coronary blood perfusion performed by hand with a conventional 5 ml plastic syringe. The blood is taken from the patient's femoral artery with the same syringe.

Results

Since January 1984 the long wire technique has been applied to more than 1000 patients. In comparison to conventional techniques, the unhindered manipulation of the wire and the optimal contrast display during the procedure have been found to be of remarkable advantage. In 13% of patients an exchange of the balloon catheter over the long wire was performed. In 5% it was necessary to use a smaller balloon diameter because crossing of the stenosis with the originally chosen catheter was not possible; in 8%, the result achieved with the first chosen catheter was not satisfactory and therefore a larger balloon was applied. In another 5% of patients, after drawback of the balloon catheter the result was not statisfactory and redilatation was performed using the same balloon catheter.

In 20 patients, branching stenoses were approached using two long guide wires. In two instances sequential dilatation was necessary; in both patients balloon expansion in one branch caused occlusion of the other. With the wire in place this occlusion could be easily passed and sequential balloon expansion performed (Fig. 4). In the majority of patients it was not necessary to introduce a balloon catheter over the second wire.

4.5% of patients showed coronary occlusion after dilatation. In the majority with the long wire in place a balloon catheter was reintroduced and another series of dilatations performed. If sufficient dilatation was not achieved,

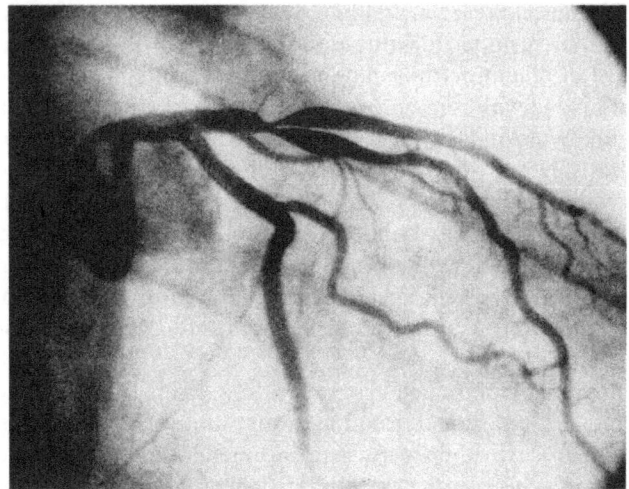

Fig. 4a. Example of branching stenosis involving the LAD and a large diagonal branch

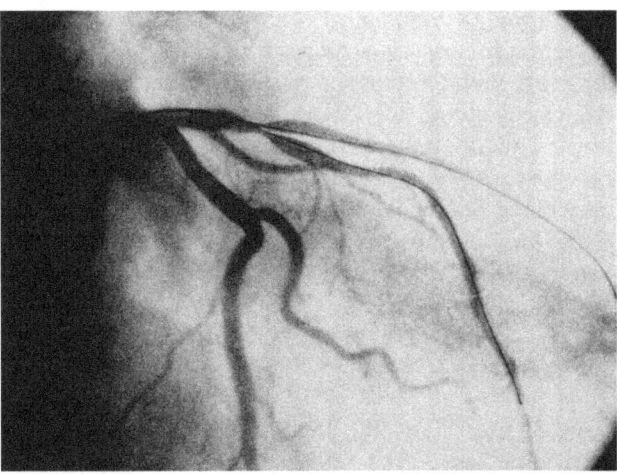

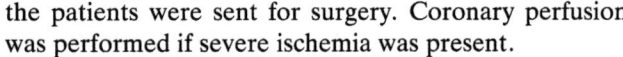

Fig. 4b. One wire in LAD and the other in the diagonal branch. After expansion of the balloon in the LAD total occlusion of the diagonal branch occurred. The balloon catheter was introduced over the second wire and expanded in the diagonal branch. A good final result was achieved

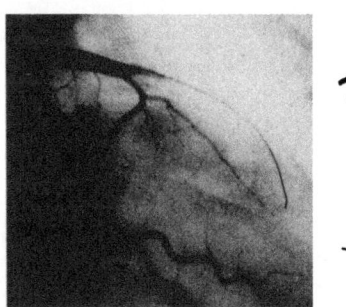 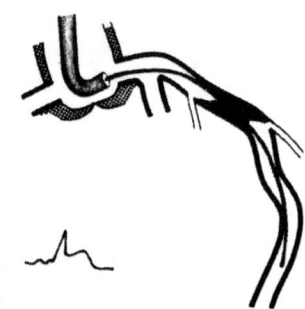

Fig. 5a. In a patient with LAD stenosis, occlusion of the LAD occurred after balloon expansion with dissection causing ST elevation and cardiogenic shock. The tip of the long wire is still in the distal LAD after the balloon catheter has been pulled back

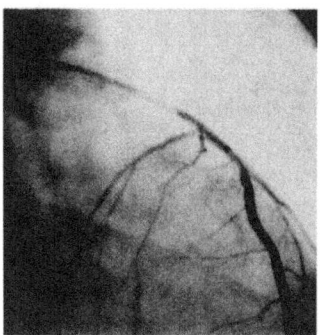

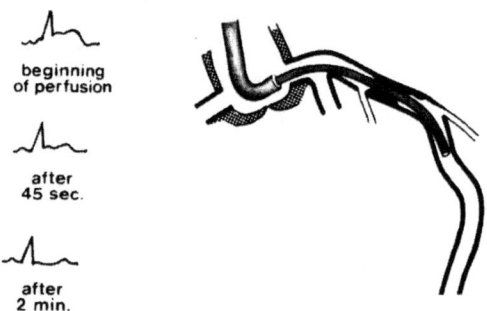

Fig. 5b. Over the long wire a 5 F perfusion catheter was introduced distal to the occlusion and the wire withdrawn. With arterial blood taken from the femoral artery intermittent perfusion was performed using a 5 ml syringe. Within 2 min the patient's condition improved, hemodynamics and the ECG normalized

the patients were sent for surgery. Coronary perfusion was performed if severe ischemia was present.

Two patients developed severe cardiogenic shock after acute coronary occlusion. The 4.5 F perfusion catheter was passed through the obstruction and the distal coronary artery was perfused with arterial blood taken from the femoral artery (Fig. 5). With perfusion of 50–100 ml/min impressive restoration of pump function was achieved. In one patient successful redilatation was performed; in the other, perfusion was continued over more than 2 h until surgical revascularization was complete.

Discussion

The free mobility of the wire and optimal contrast display during manipulation in this technique facilitate crossing of coronary stenoses. The technique allows the exchange of balloon catheters without the necessity of recrossing the stenosis with another wire. In the case of coronary obstruction, the introduction of a perfusion catheter is possible and blood perfusion of the distal coronary artery can be performed using conventional plastic syringes.

The free mobility of the wire within the guiding catheter allows an unimpeded transmission of longitudinal and rotational movements between shaft and tip of the wire. Any resistance to the tip is easily recognized and therefore the maneuver becomes extremely sensitive.

Since the wire in contrast to the balloon catheter scarcely reduces the cross sectional area of the guiding catheter, optimal contrast injections during the process of crossing are possible. All anatomical details in the area of the stenosis, as well as small side branches, and the exact positioning of the wire tip, can be recognized far better than with the usual technique.

With the long wire remaining in place, balloon exchange is possible without recrossing the stenosis. This is of help in tight stenoses, in which the first chosen balloon does not cross. Exchange of the balloon catheter and introduction of smaller sized including super-low profile balloons can be achieved without difficulty. This is possible because the 0.012″ wire also allows – in contrast to the wire extension system – the passage of very small balloon catheters. In other patients transition from a smaller to a larger balloon is necessary and easily possible.

If balloon inflation is followed by coronary dissection causing a stenosis or an occlusion, the wire offers the possibility of reintroducing the balloon catheter and repeating dilatation. If redilatation is unsuccessful, a perfusion catheter can be advanced distal to the occlusion. The single lumen of the perfusion catheter is larger than one lumen of the balloon catheter. Coronary perfusion with blood can therefore be performed without pump. The blood is taken from the femoral artery and injected into the obstructed coronary artery. With the help of a 5 ml plastic syringe a flow of 60 ml/min can be easily achieved. Perfusion is maintained until surgical revascularization is finished. We have performed successful perfusion for more than 2 h. Full heparinization is, of course, mandatory during the whole perfusion period.

During coronary dilatation the main risk arises from intimal dissection. The proximal coronary artery is particularly prone to this complication; however, dissection also occurs in both branches of the left coronary artery and the left main. Eccentric stenosis with irregular contours are a particular risk; in the individual case, however, the occurrence of a dissection cannot be predicted. Therefore the availability of a track over which the area of stenosis or occlusion can be recrossed is very valuable. Even in severe cardiogenic shock caused by dissection and coronary obstruction, the restoration of blood flow by a coronary perfusion catheter introduced over the long wire has been proved possible and has led to a dramatic improvement. The perfusion can be continued until surgical revascularization is completed.

Grüntzig introduced the "kissing balloon" technique for dilatation of branching stenoses. This technique requires two guiding catheters. With the long wire technique this type of stenosis can be approached using two wires introduced through the same guiding catheter (6, 9). The more important stenosis is first crossed with the long wire. Thereafter a second wire is placed beyond the stenosis in the less important sequence. If the first dilatation causes obstruction of the side branch, this obstruction can be recrossed over the wire in place. In the majority of patients, the balloon must not be introduced over the second wire. It remains on "standby". Since the dilatation procedure with two wires usually requires more time, it is of particular importance to use teflon-coated wires and to

emply the heparin-urokinase perfusion. Otherwise the standby wire may not allow the balloon to pass the obstruction due to fibrin coating. The wrapping of one wire over the other described by Simon with this technique (8) did not occur in our series. Since Simon did not emply heparin-urokinase perfusion, fibrin coating of the wire may have been the primary problem in his cases. On the other hand, heparin-urokinase perfusion may be recommended in all coronary angioplasty procedures. Systematic evaluation of wires after use has shown a reduction in thrombus formation. This effect was still present if teflonized wires were used instead of wires with gold surface.

Since balloon catheters also have thrombogenic properties, after angioplasty the balloon surface and/or the distal balloon catheter shaft often show thrombotic material in considerable quantities far larger than the wire. Heparin-urokinase perfusion is probably effective in reducing thrombus formation in this location too. Its general use may be justified but further studies are required.

References

1. Grüntzig A (1977) Coronary transluminal angioplasty. Circulation Suppl 84: 55–56
2. Simpson JB, Baim DS, Robert EW, Harrison DC (1982) A new catheter system for coronary angioplasty. Am J Cardiol 49: 1216–1222
3. Kober G, Vallbracht C, Lang H, Bussmann W-D, Hopf R, Kunkel B, Kaltenbach M (1985) Transluminale koronare Angioplastik 1977–1985. Erfahrungen bei 1000 Eingriffen. Radiologe 25: 346–353
4. Detre KM, Kelsey SF, NHLBI: Percutaneous transluminal coronary angioplasty registry, Bethesda, November 1983
5. Kadel C, Jonczyk C, Kaltenbach M (1987) Thrombotic deposits on angioplasty guide wires. Fifth Joint Meeting ESC, Santiago/Spain, Sept. 5–10, Abstract
6. Kaltenbach M (1984) Neue Technik zur steuerbaren Ballondilatation von Kranzgefäßverengungen. Z Kardiol 73: 669–672
7. Kaltenbach M (1984) The long wire technique – a new technique for steerable balloon catheter dilatation of coronary artery stenoses. Eur Heart J 5: 1004–1009
8. Simon R, Amende I, Herrmann G (1985) Angioplasty of coronary stenoses involving bifurcations: A new Technique. Circulation 72, Suppl III, 1596
9. Vallbracht C, Kaltenbach M, Kober G (1986) Doppel-Langdrahttechnik zur Ballondilatation von Verzweigungsstenosen. Herz/Kreisl 18: 378–382

Authors address:
Prof. Dr. med. M. Kaltenbach
Zentrum der Inneren Medizin
Abteilung für Kardiologie
Klinikum der Universität
Theodor-Stern-Kai 7
D-6000 Frankfurt am Main
West Germany

Koronarangioplastik – Ist das Rezidivrisiko am Tage des Eingriffes voraussagbar? Eine prospektive Untersuchung

C. Vallbracht, H. Klepzig jr., H. Hoin, M. Kaltenbach und G. Kober

Can restenosis be predicted immediately after coronary angioplasty?

Summary: Data from a retrospective study defining seven parameters of increased risk of restenosis after successful transluminal coronary angioplasty (high-grade stenoses, long stenoses, eccentric stenoses, use of high pressure, extended time of balloon inflation, stenoses in obese patients, stenoses in patients without a history of smoking) were fed into a computer. A discriminant analysis was made and an algorithm for prediction of restenosis was defined.

The validity of prediction was prospectively tested in 101 patients. In 80/101 (79.2%) prediction was possible; in 21/101 (20.8%) it was not possible. In 15/80 patients (18.8%) the prediction was: "restenosis probable"; in 65/80 patients (81.2%): "restenosis not probable". After 4.4 months 93/101 patients (92.1%) had an angiographic follow-up. The prediction "restenosis" proved to be correct in 13/15 patients (86.7%), and the prediction "no restenosis" was correct in 56/65 patients (86.2%).

It is concluded that in the majority of patients the risk of restenosis can be predicted immediately after the intervention.

Zusammenfassung: Die in einer retrospektiven Untersuchung definierten sieben Parameter eines erhöhten Rezidivrisikos (3 morphologische: Ausmaß der Lumeneinengung in %, Länge der Stenose in mm, Exzentrizität; 2 technische: maximaler Dilatationsdruck in bar, Dilatationsdauer in min; 2 klinische: Übergewicht, primärer Nichtraucher) wurden einer Diskriminanzanalyse unterzogen und die Möglichkeit der Vorhersage des Rezidivrisikos an 101 Patienten nach erfolgreicher Koronarangioplastik prospektiv untersucht. Bei 80 von 101 Patienten (79,2%) konnte anhand der sieben Parameter eine Vorhersage des Langzeitergebnisses am Tage der Dilatation erfolgen, bei 21 von 101 Patienten (20,8%) war eine sichere Vorhersage nicht möglich. Bei 15 von 80 Patienten lautete die Voraussage: „Rezidiv wahrscheinlich" (18,8%), bei 65 von 80 Patienten „Rezidiv unwahrscheinlich" (81,2%). Nach im Mittel 4,4 Monaten wurden 93 von 101 Patienten (92,1%) angiographisch kontrolliert.

Key words: transluminal coronary angioplasty; prediction of restenosis
Schlüsselwörter: Koronarangioplastik, Rezidivvoraussage

Die Vorhersage „Rezidiv" traf bei 13 von 15 Patienten (86,7%) zu, die Vorhersage „Kein Rezidiv" bei 58 von 65 Patienten (86,2%).

Es wird gefolgert, daß anhand dieser sieben Parameter die Vorhersage des Rezidivrisikos am Tage des Eingriffes bei der Mehrzahl der Patienten möglich ist.

Einleitung

Rezidive nach erfolgreicher Koronarangioplastik werden in großen Untersuchungsreihen mit einer Häufigkeit von 17–35% angegeben [5, 7] und stellen damit eines der ungelösten Probleme der Ballondilatation dar. Der Zeitpunkt des Rezidiveintrittes liegt ganz überwiegend innerhalb der ersten Monate nach dem Eingriff [5, 7, 10, 18]; Spätrezidive bei angiographisch dokumentiertem Erfolg mindestens 4 Monate nach dem Eingriff sind eine seltene Ausnahme [1, 2, 3, 15, 17].

Wird eine vor dem Eingriff bestehende typische Angina-pectoris-Symptomatik und eine Ischämiereaktion im Belastungs-EKG durch die Angioplastik deutlich gebessert, so kann ein Rezidiv bei etwa $^2/_3$ der Patienten am Wiederauftreten der Symptome und/oder der ischämischen ST-Strecken-Veränderungen erkannt werden (17). Bei einer kleineren Gruppe von Patienten treten jedoch trotz angiographisch gesicherter erneuter hochgradiger Stenosierung typische Symptome nicht wieder auf. Die sichere Erfolgsbeurteilung ist daher nur durch routinemäßige Kontrollangiographien 4 Monate nach dem Eingriff möglich. Da der organisatorische und zeitliche Aufwand hierfür in großen Zentren beträchtlich ist, wäre zur besseren Planung von Nachangiographien mit oder ohne Dilatationsbereitschaft und zur Vermeidung unnötiger Mehrfachangiographien eine frühzeitige Kenntnis über eine erhöhte Rezidivwahrscheinlichkeit von Bedeutung. Faktoren eines erhöhten Rezidivrisikos sind vielfach beschrieben worden [4, 5, 6, 9, 11, 12, 14, 16] und zeigen neben widersprüchlichen Befunden übereinstimmend eine besondere Bedeutung der Stenosemorphologie [6, 9, 11, 12]. In einer eigenen retrospektiven Untersuchung [18] konnten sieben Parameter definiert werden, die signifikant mit dem Auftreten von Rezidiven verbunden waren: 3 morphologische (Ausmaß der Lumeneinengung in %, Länge der Stenose in mm, Exzentrizität), 2 technische (maximaler Dilatationsdruck in bar, Dilatationsdauer in min) und 2 klinische (Übergewicht, primärer Nichtraucher).

Ziel der vorliegenden prospektiven Studie war, zu prüfen, ob anhand dieser unmittelbar nach dem Eingriff verfüg-

Tabelle 1. Untersuchung des Rezidivrisikos eingeteilt in 7 Parametern (n = 101)

Rezidivparameter	Gruppe 1 Rezidiv wahrscheinlich n = 15	Gruppe 2 Rezidiv unwahrscheinlich n = 65	Gruppe 3 Voraussage nicht möglich n = 21
Mittl. Stenosegrad vor PTCA	87,27%	80,60%	83,36%
Mittl. Stenoselänge	5,69 mm	3,08 mm	4,10 mm
Anteil exzentrischer Stenosen	12/15 (80%)	41/65 (63%)	16/21 (76%)
Mittl. maximaler Dilatationsdruck	5,89 bar	4,94 bar	6,08 bar
Mittl. Dilatationsdauer	174,3 s	154,8 s	154,1 s
Anteil der Patienten mit Übergewicht	11/15 (73,3%)	19/65 (29,2%)	9/21 (42,8%)
Anteil der primären Nichtraucher	4/15 (26,7%)	9/65 (13,8%)	6/21 (28,6%)

baren Parameter eine Voraussage des Rezidivrisikos möglich ist.

Methodik

1. Rezidivparameter

In einer vorausgegangenen retrospektiven Untersuchung wurde 62 Patienten mit angiographisch gesichertem Rezidiv entsprechend der NHLBI-Definition [5] nach erfolgreicher Angioplastik einer Einzelstenose im Sinne einer Zufallsauswahl jeweils der einem Rezidivpatienten zeitlich folgende Patient ohne Rezidiv gegenübergestellt (18). Beide Gruppen zeigten keine signifikanten Unterschiede bezüglich Alter, Geschlecht, Angina-pectoris-Dauer und -Schweregrad, Anzahl der zuvor abgelaufenen Infarkte, Anteil der Mehrgefäßerkrankungen sowie bezüglich der maximalen Größe des verwendeten Ballonkatheters und des akut erreichten Dilatationsergebnisses. Sieben Parameter waren dagegen signifikant häufer mit dem Auftreten von Rezidiven verbunden: hochgradige Stenosen vor Dilatation (86,2% vs. 82,2%; p < 0,05), langstreckige Stenosen (4,93 mm vs. 3,51 mm; p < 0,01), exzentrische Stenosen (31 vs. 16; p < 0,01), höhere maximal erforderliche Ballondrücke (6,31 bar vs. 5,68 bar; p < 0,05), längere Balloninflationszeiten (55,9 s vs. 48,9 s; p < 0,05), Übergewicht (50% vs. 24,2%; p < 0,01) und primäres Nichtrauchen (58,1% vs. 38,7%; p < 0,01).

Diese sieben Parameter der 62 Patienten mit und 62 Patienten ohne Rezidiv wurden nun einer Diskriminanzanalyse unterzogen, die zu jedem Parameter einen seiner Vorhersagewertigkeit entsprechenden Umrechnungsfaktor ergab, wobei die mit der Morphologie der Stenose verbundenen Werte den größten Vorhersagewert zeigten (Stenosegrad in % × 0,1381; Länge der Stenose in mm × 5,995; exzentrische Stenose 0,7087, konzentrische Stenose 0; max. Ballondruck in bar × 0,4271; Balloninflationszeit gesamt in Minuten × 0,0010; Übergewicht 1,6910, Normalgewicht 0; Ex-Raucher × 1,9358, primäre Nichtraucher 0). Die Addition dieser Faktoren ergab für jeden Patienten einen Zahlenwert, der eine Zuordnung in einer der drei Gruppen „Rezidiv wahrscheinlich" (Gruppe 1), „Rezidiv unwahrscheinlich" (Gruppe 2) oder „Vorhersage nicht möglich" (Gruppe 3) zuließ.

Es wurden nun Grenzwerte festgelegt, bis zu denen ein Patient mit einer theoretischen Irrtumswahrscheinlichkeit von 5% einer der drei Gruppen zugeordnet werden

konnte. Bis zu einem Zahlenwert von 15,8 wurde ein gutes Langzeitergebnis ohne Rezidiv, über 17,7 ein erhöhtes Rezidivrisiko angenommen. Werte zwischen 15,8 und 17,7 entsprachen der Grauzone, in der eine Vorhersage nicht gemacht werden konnte.

Diese retrospektiv gewonnenen Werte wurden nun durch die folgende prospektive Untersuchung geprüft.

2. Patienten

Im Zeitraum von 7/86 bis 10/86 wurden 101 konsekutive Patienten nach erfolgreicher Angioplastik einer Einzelstenose in einem nativen Koronargefäß in die Untersuchung einbezogen. Ausgeschlossen wurden 9 Patienten, bei denen nach erfolgreicher Ballondehnung der Bereich der Dilatation nicht wieder in jeder vor dem Eingriff vorliegenden Projektionsebene dargestellt worden war. Unmittelbar nach dem Eingriff wurde der oben beschriebene Zahlenwert errechnet und die Voraussage „Rezidiv wahrscheinlich", „Rezidiv unwahrscheinlich" oder „Vorhersage nicht möglich" festgelegt und verschlüsselt.

Unter den 101 Patienten befanden sich 88 Männer (87,1%) und 13 Frauen (12,9%) im Alter von 26 bis 70 Jahren (mittleres Alter 54,6 Jahre).

Bei 65 Patienten (64,4%) war die Stenose im Ramus interventricularis ant., bei 12 (11,8%) im Ramus circumflexus und bei 24 Patienten (23,8%) in der rechten Kranzarterie lokalisiert.

3. Filmauswertung

Die Angiographiefilme des Dilatationseingriffes (Kinofilm, 35 mm, 12 oder 25 Bilder pro s) wurden von zwei unabhängigen Untersuchern ausgewertet. Die Stenosierung wurde im Vergleich zu benachbarten proximalen und distalen unveränderten Arterienabschnitten in % linearer Durchmesserminderung mit Hilfe einer kleinen Schablone gemessen. Bei ungleichen Angaben der beiden Untersucher wurde der Mittelwert gebildet.

Die Länge der Stenose (gemessen wurde der hochgradige Anteil; vgl. 18) wurde gemessen und mit Hilfe des bekannten Durchmessers des Führungskatheters in mm umgerechnet (12). Eine Stenose wurde dann als exzentrisch eingestuft, wenn das Restlumen in mindestens einer Ebene ganz auf einer Seite der Mittellinie lag (12).

Als Dilatationsdruck wurde der maximal verwendete Druck in bar, als Dilatationsdauer das Produkt aus Dauer und Anzahl der Einzeldilatationen verwendet. Die Definition des Übergewichtes folgte der Broca-Regel.

4. Technik und Medikamente

Alle Eingriffe wurden mit der Langdraht-Technik nach Kaltenbach durchgeführt (8).

Während des Eingriffes wurden nach Eröffnung der Arterie 100 E/kg Körpergewicht Heparin intraarteriell als Bolus gegeben; während des Sondierungs- und Dilatationsvorganges wurde der Führungskatheter mit einer Mischung aus 2000 E Heparin und 100 000 E Urokinase pro Stunde perfundiert.

Wenigstens 24 Stunden vor, während und für die Zeit bis zur angiographischen Nachuntersuchung erhielten alle Patienten 1,5 g Acetylsalicylsäure, 2 × 50 mg Gallopamil und 60–100 mg Isosorbitdinitrat pro Tag; Betablocker wurden eine Woche vor dem Eingriff abgesetzt und nach dem Eingriff nicht wieder verordnet, um eine mögliche Erhöhung der Neigung zu Gefäßspasmen auszuschließen.

5. Zeitpunkt und Auswertung der Kontrollangiographien

Bei 93/101 Patienten (92,1%) erfolgte eine Kontrollangiographie im Mittel 17 Wochen (5 Wochen bis 9 Monate) nach dem Eingriff. Die Angiographiefilme wurden in identischen Projektionsebenen ausgewertet, die schriftlich festgelegte Vorhersage war den auswertenden Untersuchern unbekannt.

Als Rezidivdefinition wurde verwendet: „Verlust von mindestens der Hälfte des ursprünglichen Gewinns" [5].

Ergebnisse

1. Gruppenzuteilung unmittelbar nach dem Eingriff

Mit den aus der Diskriminanzanalyse gewonnenen Grenzwerten konnte bei 80 von 101 Patienten (79,2%) eine Vorhersage des Langzeitergebnisses am Tage der Dilatation erfolgen (Gruppen 1 und 2); bei 21 von 101 Patienten (20,8%) war eine ausreichend sichere Vorhersage anhand der sieben Parameter nicht möglich (Gruppe 3).

Bei 15 von 80 Patienten (18,8%) lautete die Vorhersage: „Rezidiv wahrscheinlich", bei 65 von 80 Patienten (81,2%): „Rezidiv unwahrscheinlich" (vgl. Tab. 1).

2. Ergebnisse der Nachangiographie

a) Vorhersage: Rezidiv wahrscheinlich (Gruppe 1)
15/15 Patienten (100%) wurden angiographisch kontrolliert.
13 von 15 Patienten (86,7%) wiesen ein Stenoserezidiv entsprechend der angiographischen Definition (5) auf. 2 von 15 Patienten (13,3%) waren entgegen der Vorhersage ohne Rezidiv geblieben.
Die Abbildung 1 zeigt ein Originalbeispiel mit Berechnung des Vorhersagewertes.

b) Vorhersage: Rezidiv unwahrscheinlich (Gruppe 2)
58 von 65 Patienten (89,2%) wurden angiographisch kontrolliert.
Ohne Rezidiv waren 50 von 58 Patienten geblieben (86,2%); bei 8 von 58 Patienten (13,8%) war es entgegen der Vorhersage zu einem Rückfall gekommen. Die Abbildung 2 zeigt ein Originalbeispiel.

c) Vorhersage nicht möglich (Gruppe 3)
20 von 21 Patienten (95,2%) wurden angiographisch kontrolliert.
16 von 20 Patienten (80%) zeigten ein anhaltend gutes Dilatationsergebnis, bei 4 von 20 Patienten (20%) war ein Rezidiv nachweisbar.

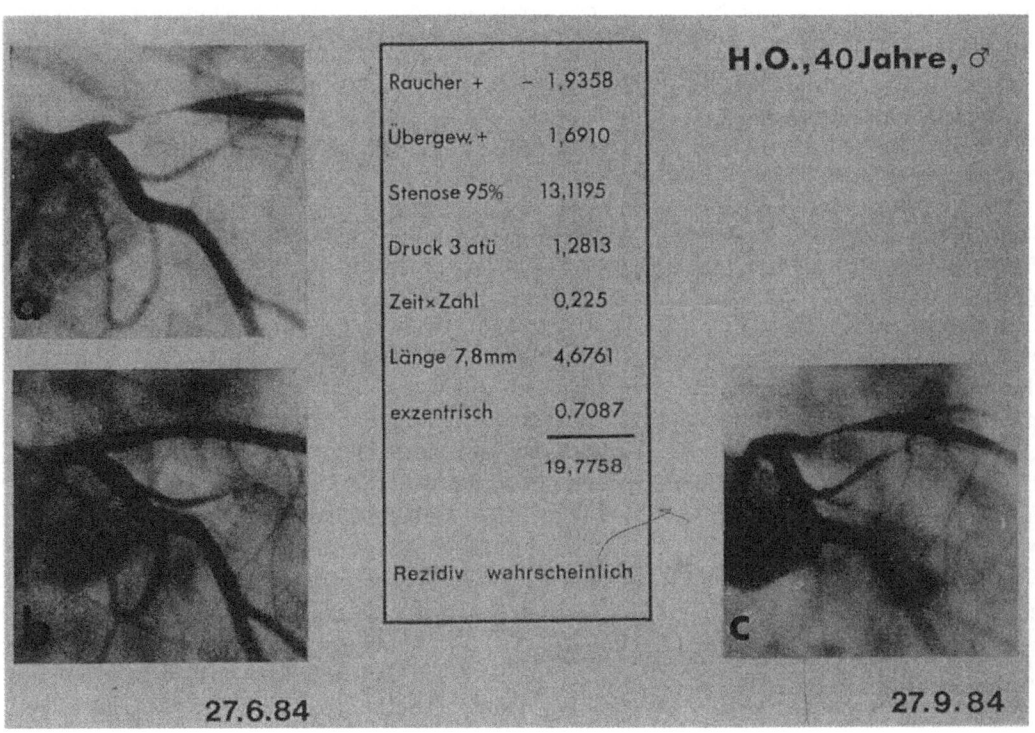

Abb. 1. Exzentrische, hochgradige und langstreckige Stenose des R. interventricularis ant. (**A**). Akutergebnis der Koronarangioplastik (**B**). Die Addition der Rezidivparameter am Tag der Dilatation ergibt die Vorhersage: Rezidiv wahrscheinlich. Die Kontrollangiographie nach 3 Monaten bestätigt den Befund einer Rezidivstenose (**C**)

Diskussion

Rezidive nach erfolgreicher transluminaler koronarer Ballondilatation stellen mit einer Häufigkeit von 17–35 % [5, 7] eines der Hauptprobleme dieser Behandlungsmethode dar.

Während weitgehende Übereinstimmung über die Behandlung der Rückfälle besteht, die in nahezu allen Fällen erneut mit der Angioplastik möglich ist und im Vergleich zum Ersteingriff höhere Akuterfolgs- und niedrigere Komplikationsraten aufweist [13], differieren die Angaben über Parameter eines erhöhten Rezidivrisikos erheblich [4, 5, 6, 9, 11, 12, 14, 16, 18]. Die Vorhersagbarkeit eines erhöhten Rückfallrisikos ist aus vielen Gründen wünschenswert (bessere Information des Patienten, Planung der Nachangiographie mit oder ohne Dilatationsbereitschaft).

Geht man davon aus, daß wie in unserem Patientengut [18] bei etwa 80 % der Patienten vor dem Eingriff eine typische Angina-pectoris-Symptomatik und/oder Ischämiereaktion im Belastungs-EKG besteht und diese wiederum bei etwa 80 % der Patienten durch den Eingriff beseitigt bzw. deutlich gebessert werden kann, so ist ein Rezidiv bei 66 % der Patienten am Wiederauftreten der Symptome zuverlässig erkennbar [17].

Die Konsequenz hieraus ist eine funktionelle Kontrolluntersuchung aller erfolgreich dilatierten Patienten etwa 2 bis 3 Wochen vor der geplanten angiographischen Nachuntersuchung. Eine funktionelle Verschlechterung gegenüber dem Akutergebnis ergibt den Verdacht auf ein Rezidiv und bedingt damit die Planung der Nachangiographie in Dilatationsbereitschaft.

Die prospektive Untersuchung der Vorhersage des Rezidivrisikos am Tage des Eingriffes zeigt, daß damit 80 % der Patienten erfaßt werden, während bei 20 % die Vorhersage nicht möglich ist. Die Vorhersage „Rezidiv wahrscheinlich" oder „Rezidiv unwahrscheinlich" trifft in jeweils mehr als 80 % zu, so daß, wiederum bezogen auf die Gesamtzahl der erfolgreich dilatierten Patienten, in erneut etwa 66 % eine relativ sichere Vorhersage des Langzeitergebnisses möglich ist.

Unmittelbar nach dem Eingriff besteht damit die Möglichkeit, mit hoher Treffsicherheit die angiographische Kontrolluntersuchung mit oder ohne Dilatationsbereitschaft zu planen, was insbesondere im Hinblick auf die eventuell notwendige Operationsbereitschaft von erheblicher Bedeutung ist.

Die Kombination der funktionellen Kontrolle mittels Belastungs-EKG 2 bis 3 Wochen vor der geplanten angiographischen Nachuntersuchung mit der Vorhersage anhand der beschriebenen 7 Parameter müßte den Anteil der voraussagbaren Rezidive noch weiter erhöhen; eine entsprechende prospektive Untersuchung mit diesem 8. Parameter wurde in Frankfurt bereits begonnen.

Weitere Untersuchungen müssen zeigen, ob es verantwortbar ist, bei Patienten, bei denen ein Rezidiv nach der oben angeführten Vorhersage und nach dem Ergebnis des Kontroll-Belastungs-EKGs weitgehend ausgeschlossen werden kann, auf eine Nachangiographie ganz zu verzichten.

Literatur

1. Grüntzig AR, Schlumpf M, Siegenthaler WE (1984) Long-term results after coronary angioplasty. Circulation 70: 323 (Suppl II)
2. Grüntzig AR, King SB III, Schlumpf M, Siegenthaler WE (1987) Long-term follow-up after percutaneous transluminal coronary angioplasty. The early Zürich experience. N Engl J Med 316/18: 1127–1132

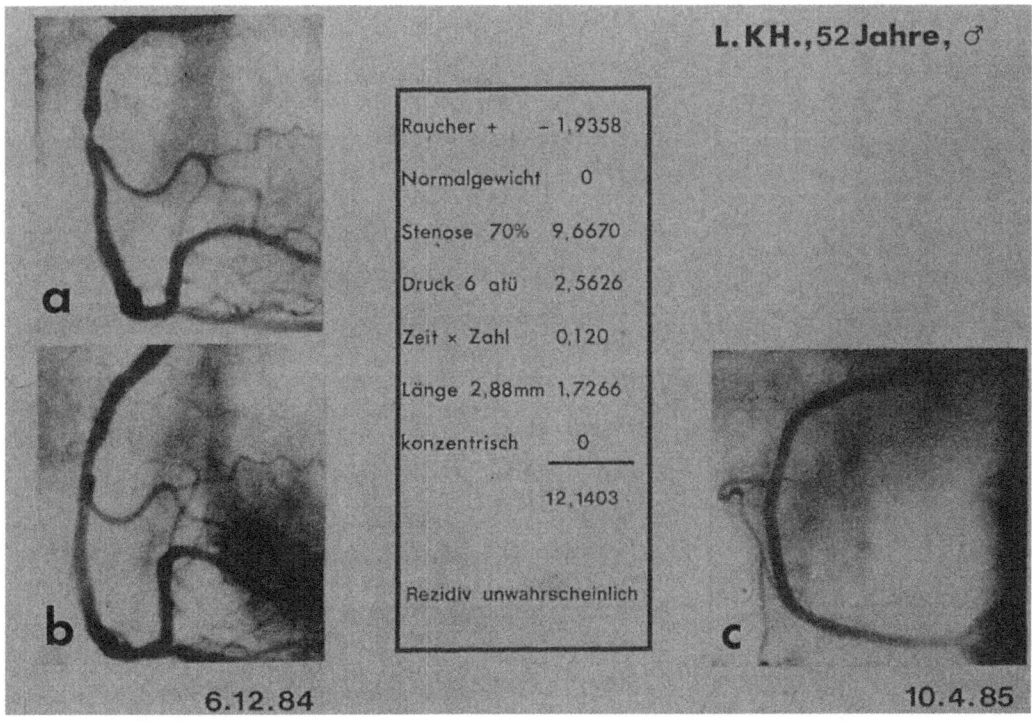

Abb. 2. Konzentrische, kurzstreckige, 70%ige Stenose der rechten Kranzarterie (**A**). Akutergebnis nach Koronarangioplastik (**B**). Die Addition der Rezidivparameter am Tag der Dilatation ergibt die Vorhersage: Rezidiv unwahrscheinlich. Die Kontrollangiographie nach 4 Monaten bestätigt das gute Langzeitergebnis (**C**).

3. Hirzel HO, Eichhorn P, Kappenberger L, Gauder MP, Schlumpf M, Grüntzig AR (1985) Percutaneous transluminal coronary angioplasty: Late results at 5 year following intervention. Am Heart J 109, No 3: 575–581

4. Holmes DR, Vlietstra RE, Smith HC, Vetrovec GW, Cowley MJ, Kent KM, Dentre KR, Myler R (1982) Restenosis following percutaneous transluminal coronary angioplasty (PTCA): a report from the NHLBI, PTCA registry. Am J Cardiol 49: 905

5. Holmes DR, Vlietstra RE, Smith HC, Vetrovec GW, Kent KM, Cowley MJ, Faxon DP, Grüntzig A, Kelsey SF, Dentre KM (1984) Restenosis after percutaneous transluminal coronary angioplasty (PTCA): a report from the PTCA registry of the NHLBI. Am J Cardiol 53: 77c–81c

6. Ischinger T, Grüntzig A, Hollman J, King SB III, Douglas J, Meier B, Bradford J, Tankersley R (1983) Should coronary arteries with less than 60% diameter stenosis be treated with angioplasty? Circulation 68: 148–154

7. Kaltenbach M, Kober G, Scherer D, Vallbracht C (1984) Rezidivhäufigkeit nach erfolgreicher Ballondilatation von Kranzarterienstenosen. Z Kardiol 73 (Suppl 2): 161–166

8. Kaltenbach M (1984) Neue Technik zur steuerbaren Ballondilatation von Kranzgefäßverengungen. Z Kardiol 73: 669–673

9. Lamberto G, Bentivoglio JM, Raden JV, Sheryle F, Kelsey PhD, Dentre M (1984) Percutaneous transluminal coronary angioplasty (PTCA) in patients with relative contraindications: Results of the NHLBI PTCA registry. Am J Cardiol 53: 82c–88c

10. Leimgruber PP, Roubin GS, Hollman J, Cotsonis GA, Meier B, Douglas JS, King SB III, Grüntzig A (1985) Restenosis after successful coronary angioplasty in patients with single vessel disease. Circulation 73: 710–717

11. Marantz T, Williams DO, Reiner S, Gerwitz H, Most AS (1984) Predictors of restenosis after successful coronary angioplasty. Circulation (Suppl II) 70: 710

12. Meier B, Grüntzig AR, Hollman J, Ischinger T, Bradford JM (1983) Does length or eccentricity of coronary stenoses influence the outcome of transluminal dilatation? Circulation 67: 497–499

13. Meier B, King SB III, Grüntzig AR, Douglas JS, Hollmann J, Ischinger Y, Galan K, Tankersley R (1984) Repeat coronary angioplasty. J Amer Coll Cardiol 4: 463–466

14. Meyer J, Schmitz H, Erbel R, Böcker-Josephs B, Grenner H, Krebs W, Merx W, Bardos P, Messmer BJ, Minale C, Effert S (1982) Transluminal angioplasty in patients with unstable angina pectoris. In: Kaltenbach M, Grüntzig A, Rentrop K, Bussmann WD (eds) Transluminal coronary angioplasty and intracoronary thrombolysis. Springer-Verlag, Heidelberg New York, pp 367–371

15. Rosing DR, Cannon RO III, Watson RM, Bonow RO, Mincemeyer R, Ewels C, Leon MB, Lakatsos E, Epstein SE, Kent KM (1987) Three year anatomic, functional and clinical follow-up after successful percutaneous transluminal coronary angioplasty. JAAC Vol 9: 1–7

16. Scholl JM, David PR, Chaitman BR, Lesperance J, Cipeau J, Dydra J, Bourassa MG (1981) Recurrence of stenosis following percutaneous transluminal coronary angioplasty. Circulation (Suppl IV) 64: 193

17. Vallbracht C, Hermansson S, Kober G, Kaltenbach M, Schütz J (1987) Angiographische und funktionelle Langzeitergebnisse 2–8 Jahre nach Koronarangioplastik. Z Kardiol 76: 713–717

18. Vallbracht C, Klepzig H jr, Giesecke A, Kaltenbach M, Kober G (1987) Transluminale koronare Angioplastik: Parameter eines erhöhten Rezidivrisikos. Z Kardiol 76: 727–732

Recognition of Restenosis: Can Patients be Defined in Whom the Exercise-ECG Result Makes Angiographic Restudy Unnecessary?

C. Kadel, T. Strecker, M. Kaltenbach and G. Kober

The value of exercise ECG in predicting the occurrence of restenosis after successful transluminal coronary angioplasty (PTCA) was investigated in 398 patients with exercise tests of comparable workload before, immediately after and within 6 months after PTCA. In patients with normalized exercise ECG (n = 166) restenosis was observed in 16.3% and indication for repeat PTCA was present in 6.6%. RePTCA was recommended in only 3.2% of patients if the exercise test was still normal at restudy and if the patients were free of anginal symptoms. In patients with a renewed ST-segment depression (n = 77) the rate of restenosis was 67.5% and the indication for rePTCA was present in 52%. In patients without changes in the exercise tests before and after PTCA and at restudy (n = 155) restenosis was seen in 25.8% and rePTCA was recommended in 14.2%. It is concluded that from the clinical point of view, in patients with improved exercise ECG at restudy, especially if they are free of angina, there is no need for a re-angiogram because indications for rePTCA are very rare.

Introduction

After more than 10 years' experience in PTCA, restenosis is still a major unsolved problem. Restenosis develops in 15–40% of all successfully dilated patients [1–4], in almost every case within 6 months of the procedure. Most patients with a severe restenosis undergo repeat PTCA. Although several predictors of restenosis are known [5, 6], until now there has been no generally accepted therapeutic method to reduce the rat of restenosis significantly.

With the increasing number of patients undergoing PTCA there is also an increasing need for follow-up procedures that identify patients with restenoses. The 'gold standard' in the determination of restenosis is still the coronary angiogram, but there are several non-invasive methods available, such as exercise ECG, thallium scintigraphy and radionuclide ventriculography, which can be applied for the evaluation of the immediate and long-term functional success after PTCA [7–14]. The advantage of the exercise ECG especially is that it can be repeatedly performed even in unspecialized centres without much risk and discomfort for the patient.

Thus it was the aim of this study to investigate the value of exercise ECG in defining a group of patients who do not need angiographic restudy after successful PTCA.

Patients and methods

Between 1982 and 1987, 587 patients had successful PTCA and follow-up angiogram at our hospital. 398 of these patients with three exercise ECGs at comparable workloads were included in this study. The first exercise ECG was performed within 7 days before PTCA, the second within 3 days after PTCA and the third ≤ 7 days before the repeat angiogram. The patients' baseline data are shown in Table 1.

Indications for PTCA were a diameter stenosis of 70% or more suitable for PTCA, evidence of ischaemia on exercise ECG, thallium scintigraphy or radionuclide ventriculography and/or anginal symptoms.

Table 1. Baseline data of the patients

Males	89.4%
Females	10.6%
Single-vessel disease	75.6%
Multivessel disease	24.4%
Myocardial infarction prior to PTCA	50.8%
Dilated vessel: LAD	71.9%
RCA	16.8%
CX	8.8%
Bypass graft	1.7%
Left main stem	0.8%
Complete revascularization	67.8%

Table 2. Definition of groups

ST-segment depression	Before PTCA	After PTCA	At re-study	n
Group 1	+	−	−	130
(expected success)	+	+	−	36
Group 2	+	−	+	66
(expected restenosis)	−	−	+	11
Group 3	−	−	−	88
(uncertain outcome)	+	+	+	63
	−	+	−	3
	−	+	+	1

Positive exercise ECG: +
Negative exercise ECG: −

Key words: PTCA, restenosis, exercise ECG

Reprint from Eur. Heart J. (1989) 10 (Suppl. G.) 22–26, Academic Press, London

Acute success was defined according to NHLBI criteria as a reduction in stenosis diameter of at least 20% (estimate visually) and the absence of major complications such as myocardial infarction, emergency bypass surgery or death.

Repeat angiograms were routinely performed in all successfully dilated patients 128 ± 40 days after PTCA. Cine films were evaluated by two independent investigators. Restenosis was defined according to the NHLBI definitions as (1) loss of at least 50% of the gain achieved by PTCA and/or (2) stenosis at follow-up less than 20% wider than before PTCA and/or (3) increase in stenosis diameter of at least 30% at follow-up compared with the initial result. According to these definitions restenosis was found in 29.9% of all patients included in this study.

Exercise ECG was performed as previously described [15] in the upright position with a constantly maintained submaximal workload over 6 minutes. Exercise tests were terminated if severe angina or ST-segment depression of more than 0.3 mV occurred.

According to the results of the exercise ECG before, immediately after and 4–6 months after PTCA, patients were classified into three groups (Table 2). Group 1 includes patients with ST-segment depression before PTCA but not at restudy. Group 2 includes patients without ST-segment depression immediately after PTCA but signs of myocardial ischaemia at restudy. The third group consists of patients with any other combination. In general, no ECG change was observed during the three stress tests in these patients. To exclude any influences of untreated diseased vessels in patients with multivessel disease, subset analysis was performed for the patients with single-vessel disease within these groups. Additionally, comparable evaluations were made for patients with complete revascularization and for patients without previous myocardial infarction.

Statistical analyses were performed using the two-tailed Mann-Whitney test. Results are expressed as the mean ± 1 SD or percentage.

Results

In group 1 (patients with exercise-induced ST-segment depression before PTCA but not at restudy) a restenosis was observed in 16.3%, but only in 4.8% was the restenosis severe (> 70% in diameter reduction). 6.6% of group 1 patients were redilated due to the severity of restenosis or progression of coronary heart disease in a segment formerly not dilated (Table 3). In group 2 (patients with no ST-segment depression immediately after PTCA but with ST-segment depression at re-evaluation) a restenosis was seen in 67.5%. In 1.3% a new high-grade stenosis was detected. Indications for rePTCA were present in 52.0% (Table 3), in patients with uncertain outcome on ECG (group 3) a restenosis occurred in 25.8% and in 14.2% rePTCA was recommended (Table 3).

The mean stenosis diameter observed immediately before and after PTCA and at the date of reevaluation is shown in Table 4 for patients of group 1 and 2. The mean stenosis

Table 3. Angiographic results and therapeutic consequences of the repeat angiogram in all patients

	n	Restenosis (%)	Restenosis > 70% (%)	New stenosis > 70% (%)	re PTCA (%)
Group 1	166	16.3	4.8	0.6	6.6
Group 2	77	67.5	45.5	1.3	52.0
Group 3	155	25.8	12.9	1.3	14.2

Table 4. Stenosis diameter

	n	Pre PTCA	Post PTCA	Restudy
Group 1 (no restenosis)	139	84.3 ± 9.0	29.2 ± 12.6	29.8 ± 13.7
Group 1 (restenosis)	27	85.7 ± 9.3	33.3 ± 13.9	68.5 ± 17.5
Group 2 (no restenosis)	25	83.8 ± 8.2	31.2 ± 15.4	44.6 ± 20.7
Group 2 (restenosis)	52	83.7 ± 9.4	31.5 ± 13.5	78.5 ± 15.1

Data are $\% \pm$ SD.

diameter was 84% before and 29% after PTCA. In group 2 patients with ST-segment depression at restudy, but without restenosis according to the used definition, a small but significant increase in stenosis from 31% after PTCA to 45% at restudy was observed ($P = 0.015$).

In Table 5, the results of patients with single-vessel disease are shown. There are no major differences compared with the complete study populations of groups 1–3. Table 6 shows the results of the patients in whom a complete revascularization had been achieved by PTCA (no remaining stenosis > 50% after PTCA), and Table 7 shows the results in patients without prior myocardial infarction. Again there are no major differences to the results obtained in the complete groups 1–3.

When anginal symptoms and the exercise test were evaluated simultaneously, patients with exercise-induced ST-segment depression before PTCA, without signs of ischaemia, and no anginal symptoms during the exercise ECG at restudy showed a restenosis in 12.6%. Only 3.2% of these patients presented with restenosis > 70% diameter reduction, which was an indication for repeat PTCA. On the other hand, restenosis was seen in 76.9% of all patients with recurrent signs of ischaemia and anginal symptoms at restudy. Here the indication for repeated PTCA was present in 65.4% (Table 8).

Discussion

Successfully perfomed PTCA results in an improvement in anginal symptoms and exercise tolerance immediately after the procedure. Especially after a complete revascularization, a previously positive exercise ECG returns

Table 5. Angiographic results and therapeutic consequences of the repeat angiogram in patients with single-vessel disease

	n	Restenosis (%)	Restenosis > 70% (%)	New stenosis > 70% (%)	re PTCA (%)
Group 1	142	14.1	4.2	0.7	6.4
Group 2	56	66.1	46.4	1.8	50.0
Group 3	103	27.2	12.6	1.0	12.6

Table 6. Angiographic results and therapeutic consequences of the repeat angiogram in patients with complete revascularization

	n	Restenosis (%)	Restenosis > 70% (%)	New stenosis > 70% (%)	re PTCA (%)
Group 1	129	14.0	4.7	0	6.2
Group 2	48	70.8	47.9	0	56.3
Group 3	93	23.7	11.8	1.1	10.8

Table 7. Angiographic results and therapeutic consequences of the repeat angiogram in patients without prior myocardial infarction

	n	Restenosis (%)	Restenosis > 70% (%)	New stenosis > 70% (%)	re PTCA (%)
Group 1	78	11.5	2.6	0	5.1
Group 2	50	68.0	42.0	2.0	48.0
Group 3	68	29.4	11.8	1.5	11.8

Table 8. Angiographic results and therapeutic consequences of the repeat angiogram according to ST-segment depression and anginal symptoms during exercise ECG at restudy

	n	Restenosis (%)	Restenosis > 70% (%)	New stenosis > 70% (%)	re PTCA (%)
Group 1, no anginal symptoms	127	12.6	3.2	0.8	3.2
Group 2 anginal symptoms	52	76.9	55.8	1.9	65.4
All other patients	219	28.8	13.7	0.9	16.0

to normal. Therefore, appearance of symptoms or exercise-induced ST-segment depression within a few months after an initial improvement is very likely caused by a restenosis.

In this study, the rate of restenosis according to the NHLBI definition, the rate of severe restenosis (diameter stenosis > 70%) and the percentage of indications for

repeat PTCA was determined in 398 patients who had repeat angiogram at our hospital and stress tests a comparable workloads before, immediately after and within 6 months of PTCA. Patients included in this study were not representative of all patients treated within this time. They represented a negative selection, because symptom-free patients were more frequently restudied in outside hospitals where angioplasty for restenosis could not be performed. This selection is illustrated by the mean rate of restenosis of 30% in this study, compared with our overall rate of restenosis of 20%.

Patients with improved exercise ECG immediately after PTCA and with no ST-segment depression at re-evaluation were not expected to have restenosis. Nevertheless, in this group, repeat angiograms showed restenosis in 16% and severe restenosis in 5%. Indications for repeated PTCA was given in 7% of this group. False-negative results in these patients may be due to a training effect. It is also important that, in group 1 patients with restenoses, mean diameter reduction at re-evaluation was less than before PTCA (69% vs 86%). If only patients free of anginal complaints and with improved exercise test at restudy are taken into account rePTCA was indicated in only 3%.

These data suggest, along with the very good long-term prognosis of patients selected for PTCA [16–18], that there is no urgent indication for repeat angiograms in patients with lasting improvement of exercise ECG after PTCA, especially if they are free of anginal symptoms.

On the other hand, in patients with a previously positive exercise ECG which returns to normal immediately after PTCA and deteriorates again within the following 6 months, a restenosis is very likely the cause [9]. In these patients a restenosis was seen in 68% and repeat PTCA was performed in 52%. If patients were complaining additionally of anginal symptoms at restudy, the rate of restenosis was even higher, at 77%, and indication for rePTCA was present in 65%.

The reappearance of ST-segment depression in group 2 patients without restenosis at angiographic restudy may be partly explained by a slight but significant increase in the mean diameter reduction from 31% immediately after PTCA to 45% at restudy.

In patients without significant changes in exercise ECG immediately after the procedure and at reevaluation 3–4 months later compared with prePTCA stress test, the results of additional thallium scintigraphy and/or radionuclide ventriculography are of value in predicting restenosis, provided that a comparable investigation had been done before PTCA.

Although the result of the exercise ECG is influenced by a previous myocardial infarction [19], by the completeness of revascularization achieved by PTCA and the number of diseased vessels [8], there were no major differences observed when these parameters were taken into account in subgroups of patients.

Several predictors of restenosis are known, such as the diameter of stenosis before PTCA, length of stenosis or discontinued medical treatment [5, 6]. In a prospective study, prediction of patients free of restenosis at follow-up, considering these parameters, was correct in 86% of cases [20]. If the results of exercise ECG are taken into account, then their predictive values may be even higher.

References

1. Kaltenbach M, Kober G, Scherer D, Vallbracht C. Recurrence rate after successful coronary angioplasty. Eur Heart J 1985; 6: 276.
2. Leimgruber PP, Roubin GS, Hollman J et al. Restenosis after successful coronary angioplasty in patients with single vessel disease. Circulation 1986; 73: 710.
3. Holmes DR, Vlietstra RE, Smith HC et al. Restenosis after percutaneous transluminal coronary angioplasty (PTCA): A report from the PTCA registry of the National Heart, Lung and Blood Institute. Am J Cardiol 1984; 53: 77C.
4. Levine S. Ewels CJ, Rosing DR, Kent KM. Coronary angioplasty: Clinical and angiographic follow-up. Am J Cardiol 1985; 55: 673.
5. Vallbracht C, Klepzig H Jr., Giesecke A, Kaltenbach M, Kober G. Transluminale koronare Angioplastik: Parameter eines erhöhten Rezidivrisikos. Z Kardiol 1987: 76: 727.
6. Rapold HJ, David PR, Val PG, Mata Al, Crean PA, Bourassa MG. Restenosis and its determinants in first and repeat coronary angioplasty. Eur Heart J 1987; 8: 575.
7. Meier B, Gruentzig AR, Siegenthaler WE, Schlumpf M. Long-term exercise performance after percutaneous transluminal coronary angioplasty and coronary artery bypass grafting. Circulation 1983; 68: 796.
8. Thomas ES, Most AS, Williams DO. Objective assessment of coronary angioplasty for multivessel disease: Results of exercise stress testing. J Am Coll Cardiol 1988; 11: 217.
9. Scholl JM, Chaitman BR, David PR et al. Exercise electrocardiography and myocardial scintigraphy in the serial evaluation of the results of percutaneous transluminal coronary angioplasty. Circulation 1982; 66: 380.
10. Rosing DR, Van Raden MJ, Mincemoyer RM et al. Exercise, electrocardiographic and functional responses after percutaneous transluminal coronary angioplasty. Am J Cardiol 1984: 53: 36C.
11. Hirzel HO, Nuesch K, Gruentzig A, Luetolf UM. Short- and long-term changes in myocardial perfusion after percutaneous transluminal coronary angioplasty assessed by thallium-201 exercise scintigraphy. Circulation 1981; 63: 1001.
12. De Puey EG, Leathermann LL, Leachman RD et al. Restenosis after transluminal coronary angioplasty detected with exercise-gated radionuclide ventriculography. J Am Coll Cardiol 1984; 6: 1103.
13. Grenz R, Maul FD, Standke R, Klepzig H Jr, Kober G, Hör G. Ergebnisse der kombinierten Myokardszintigraphie und Radionuklidventrikulographie vor und nach transluminaler Koronarangioplastik kritischer Koronararterienstenosen. Nucl Med 1986; 25: 106.
14. Hör G, Kober G, Maul FD et al. Nuclear cardiology results before and after percutaneous transluminal coronary angioplasty (PTCA). Nucl Med Comm 1987: 8: 127.
15. Kaltenbach M. Exercise testing of cardiac patients. Bern, Stuttgart, Vienna, 1976.
16. Ernst SM, Van der Feltz T, Bal ET et al. Long term angiographic follow-up, cardiac events and survival in patients undergoing percutaneous transluminal coronary angiplasty. Br Heart J 1987; 57: 220.
17. Talley JD, Hurst JW, King III SB et al. Clinical outcome 5 years after attempted percutaneous transluminal angioplasty in 427 patients. Circulation, 1988; 77: 820.
18. Kadel C, Richter J, Klepzig H Jr, Kober G, Kaltenbach M. Incidence of coronary death, myocardial infarction and anginal symptoms in 837 patients with 2–9 year follow-up after PTCA. Eur Heart J, 1987; 8, Suppl 2: 249 (abstr).
19. Pellinen TJ, Virtanen KS, Valle M, Frick MH. Studies on ergometer testing II. Effect of previous myocardial infarction, digoxin and β-blockade on exercise electrocardiography. Clin Cardiol, 1986; 9: 499.
20. Vallbracht C, Klepzig H Jr, Hoin H, Kober G, Kaltenbach M. Can restenosis be predicted immediately after coronary angioplasty? (unpublished).

Results of Repeat Angiography up to Eight Years Following Percutaneous Transluminal Angioplasty

G. KOBER, C. VALLBRACHT, C. KADEL and M. KALTENBACH

Percutaneous transluminal coronary angioplasty (PTCA) has become a widely accepted procedure that provides acute and medium-term relief of anginal symptoms and myocardial ischaemia.

The acute success rate has risen from about 50% in the early days to approximately 90% in recent years. Serial repeat angiograms obtained in different patient groups have shown a 20% incidence of angiographically defined restenoses in patients who had been successfully treated initially. Despite the restenosis, many of these patients were symptomatically improved since the lesions shown at follow-up angiography were often less severe than those that had existed prior to original PTCA.

These figures suggest that a success rate of 80% at 1 year should now be a realistic expectation, especially when patients with repeat PTCA are included.

None of the 87 patients re-angiographed between 2 and 8 years after successful PTCA developed restenosis after the first year of treatment. However, new stenoses of 50% or more were found in other vessel segments, in both symptomatic and asymptomatic patients, at a rate of about 7% per year.

Introduction

It is now well established that percutaneous transluminal coronary angioplasty (PTCA) can acutely relieve anginal symptoms and myocardial ischaemia and restore a normal pattern of coronary anatomy. However, much less is known about the medium-term results of PTCA, and our knowledge of the long-term results (after several years) is also extremely limited.

In order to discuss genuinely the long-term success and restenosis rates after PTCA, it is necessary to perform repeated angiography several months and years following the initial procedure. This paper provides angiographic data obtained from different groups of patients successfully treated, who were followed up with serial angiography ≤ 8 years following the initial procedure.

Methods and patients

PTCA was introduced early in this centre. The first case was treated in October 1977. During the early years, two studies were performed in order to obtain follow-up angiographic data at 3 months and 12 months following successful procedures. The percentage diameter stenosis was ascertained by visual assessment in the first (retro-spective) study (Group 1), and by using caliper measurements in the second (prospective) study (Group 2). Success and restenosis rates were determined using NIH-defined criteria [5]. Any angiogram that satisfied at least one of the NIH criteria was considered to show restenosis. 'Maintenance of ≥ 20% improvement' correlated best with the clinical outcome [17].

All coronary angiograms (initial and repeat) were acquired after routine administration of 0.8 mg nitroglycerin sublingually. In order to facilitate comparisons between different angiograms of the same patient, similar projections were used. Patients were given aspirin (1.5 g daily), verapamil (80 mg t.i.d.) or gallopamil (50 mg b.i.d. or t.i.d.) and ISDN (20 mg t.i.d.) for at least 2 days prior to PTCA. If this regimen was well tolerated, it was continued until the re-angiography 3–5 months following the initial procedure. Whenever possible, patients thereafter continued on aspirin and calcium blockers; ISDN was discontinued only in asymptomatic patients.

The follow-up data of the first 356 cases successfully treated by PTCA (Group I) were analysed retrospectively [7]. A total of 439 angiograms were obtained. Of the 356 patients initially treated, 333 (94%) were re-angiographed at least once; 311 patients (87%) underwent repeat angiography at 3 months; Restenosis was found in 61, leaving 295 of whom 122 (41%) were re-angiographed again at 12 months after the initial procedure. The 6% of patients who were not followed up by repeat angiography had refused consent and were asymptomatic.

In a second study, acute success rate, long-term success rate and complication rate were studied prospectively in 482 patients (Group II) recruited between October 1, 1981 and March 31, 1984. Repeat angiographies were obtained in 94% of the 345 successfully treated cases (acute success rate: 71.6%); angiograms were acquired after 18 weeks in 93%, and again after 66 weeks in 80% of cases. The total number of repeat angiograms was 598. For a total of 87 unselected patients who underwent PTCA between 1977 and 1985, long-term angiographic data, covering a post-PTCA period of two or more years, are now available. 81 of these patients have been re-angiographed < 1 year after PTCA. Late angiography was performed between 2 and 3 years after PTCA in 30% of cases, and within 8 years of the initial procedure in the

Key words: Coronary angioplasty, recurrence rate, new stenoses, long-term follow-up angiography.

Reprint from Eur. Heart J. (1989) 10 (Suppl. G.) 49–53, Academic Press, London

Table 1. Chronology of long-term angiographic follow-up after successful angioplasty (1978–1985)

	Number (%) of patients
Angiography due to symptoms	65
Angiography without symptoms	22
2–3 years following PTCA	26 (30)
3–4 years following PTCA	33 (38)
4–5 years following PTCA	19 (22)
5–6 years following PTCA	5 (6)
6–8 years following PTCA	4 (5)

Among 87 successfully TCA-treated patients with follow-up angiograms ≥2 years after angioplasty, 65 (75%) had angina pectoris, 22 (25%) did not

remaining patients (Table 1). At the time of late angiography, 22 patients were asymptomatic while 65 had had a recurrence of anginal symptoms.

Results

Group I patients (Table 2)

Of the 356 patients successfully treated with PTCA, 87% were re-angiographed at 3 months; 41% of those who had no evidence of restenosis at that time underwent repeat angiography 12 months after the initial procedure. The overall recurrence rate was 17%. Where PTCA had been performed on native vessels, the recurrence rate was even lower, at 15.4%.

Group II patients (Table 3)

In this prospective study, 21% (69 out of 345 successfully treated patients) had a recurrence of the original stenosis within a mean of 66 weeks. 64% of these patients underwent repeat PTCA with an acute success rate of 90% and long-term success rate of 73%. Thus, the 66-week success rate for all patients in this study group amounted to 63.5%, taking into account the acute success rate of 71.6% of the initial procedure and the results of re-PTCA (Table 4).

However, the long-term success rate of the group of patients with an initially successful PTCA was 88.7%.

Data on long-term follow-up angiography covering a post-PTCA period of ≥ 2 years are available for 87 patients (mean follow-up of 3.6 years). Within the group as a whole, 81 patients were re-angiographed in the first year after PTCA (Fig. 1). Of the 69 patients whose early repeat angiograms had not shown any signs of restenosis, none had evidence of late stenosis between 2 and 8 years. Equally no late restenosis was observed in three patients with early recurrence who were successfully redilated; neither was there late restenosis in the six patients who had not undergone early re-angiography. Nine patients had evidence of restenosis on the early repeat angiograms but were not invasively managed; of these, two suffered a further progression of their lesions resulting in 100% and 90% luminal diameter reduction, respectively. In two

Table 2. Recurrence rate after successful coronary angioplasty

Number of angiograms	Months after angioplasty	Recurrence
311	3	14%
122	12	3%
6	24–48	–
439 angiograms among 356 patients		17%
(without bypass-stenoses and recurrences)		15.4%

Angiographic follow-up in 94% (333/356) of successfully PTCA-treated patients showed a total of 17% restenosis. Recurrence rate in native vessels was 15.4%

Table 3. Long-term results of coronary angioplasty

482 patients	
Success rate (345 patients)	71.6%
Re-angiography 1 to 2 in 325/345 patients (total of 598 re-angiograms)	94.0%
Recurrence rate (mean 18 weeks)	19.5%
Recurrence rate (mean 66 weeks)	21.2%

Restenoses developed in the majority of cases within a mean of 18 weeks (19.5%), at ≤66 weeks of follow-up only an additional 1.7% were detected

Table 4. Success rate of angioplasty after 66-weeks follow-up

Acute success rate	71.6%
66-weeks success rate (including repeat TCA)	
all patients attempted	63.5%
successfully treated patients	88.7%
Anticipated long-term success rate (acute success rate 90%)	
all patients attempted	79.8%
successfully treated patients	>90.0%

Observed and anticipated acute and long-term success rates of PTCA

patients the lesions remained unchanged; and a total of five patients showed a regression of the stenosis to 31% diameter. In no case did a restenosis occur at a successfully treated site >1 year following PTCA.

Of the 87 patients that could be followed up over several years, 38 (44%) developed significant stenoses in other vessel segments (Fig. 2). Twenty of these 38 (53%) were again managed successfully with PTCA; one patient received a bypass while 17 patients were managed medically.

Discussion

PTCA has established itself as the procedure of choice for the treatment of fixed coronary artery obstructions, the improvement of coronary blood flow, and the relief of myocardial ischaemia and anginal symptoms at rest and during exercise.

Greater operator experience and more sophisticated equipment have led to dramatic improvements in the acute results, even though the cases now referred for

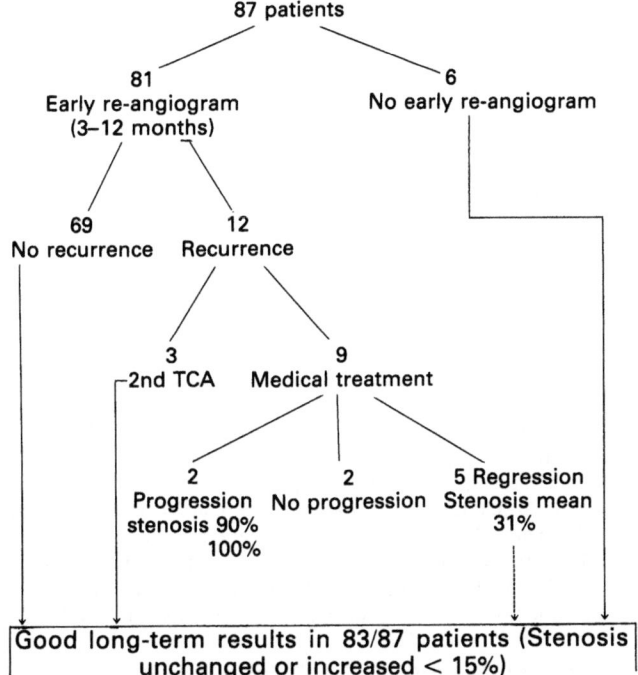

Fig. 1. Long-term angiographic follow-up in 87 patients showed no case of development of a restenosis >1 year after angioplasty

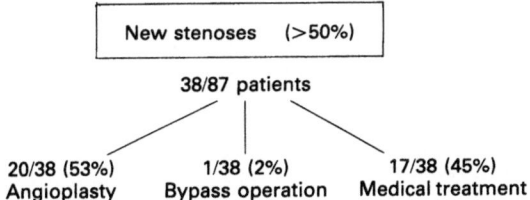

Fig. 2. Development of new stenosis and further treatment in patients 2–8 (mean 3.6) years following successful angioplasty (87 patients)

treatment tend to be anatomically more and more demanding. Thus, the acute success rate has risen from just over 50% to about 90% [1, 2, 6–10, 12]. However, our knowledge of the long-term course of PTCA-treated patients is still inadequate.

The angiographic follow-up data presented here come from different patient groups that were extensively followed up with repeat angiography (>90% at 12–18 weeks; 80% after a mean of 66 weeks), and show a total local restenosis rate of about 20% using the commonly accepted NIH criteria. This restenosis rate is low compared with the ≥30% usually reported in current literature [2, 14]. At present, no conclusive explanation can be offered to account for this discrepancy. It must be borne in mind that the restenosis rate is determined by a variety of factors, such as patient selection (stable/unstable angina), the pattern of the lesion (diameter, length, eccentricity, calcifications, etc.), technical aspects of PTCA (ratio of balloon and artery diameters; number and duration of inflations, etc.), medication before, during and after PTCA (nitrates, calcium blockers, ASA, heparin,

urokinase), and management of risk factors [2, 11, 12, 16].

Furthermore, restenosis rates can be determined only from complete, or almost complete, repeat angiographic data. The rather high restenosis rates reported by some authors may well be due, firstly, to a very limited repeat angiography rate and, secondly, to the selection of symptomatic patients for repeat angiography, thus falsely increasing the restenosis rate [4, 5, 11, 15].

Patients with a successful initial PTCA who subsequently suffer early restenosis can be managed with a second PTCA, with a high probability of a successful outcome and with little risk.

The figures quoted above show that 36% of the patients in our second (prospective) study who developed restenosis did not undergo another PTCA; this was due partly to difficulties during the original procedure (at a time when the technique was not as well controlled as it is today), and partly to the fact that the recurring lesions were fairly low-grade. The angiographic definition of restenosis comprises luminal diameter reductions by 60%, 50% and even less, i.e. lesions that are not haemodynamically significant, and which can typically be found in patients who are improved or totally asymptomatic.

Considering the low acute success rate of 71.6% achieved in the early years, and taking into account the recurrence rate after initial PTCA and repeat PTCA, as well as the success rate of repeat PTCA, 63.5% of all patients in whom PTCA was attempted showed medium-term improvement, whereas the medium-term success rate was 88.7% in those cases with a successful initial procedure. Assuming an acute success rate of 90% (to reflect what may realistically be expected nowadays), the 66-week medium-term success rate of all patients in whom PTCA was attempted would be approximately 80%, and the medium-term success rate of initially successfully treated patients would be ≥90% since repeat PTCA is now being done more often in cases of restenosis (Table 4).

In the angiographic follow-up studies, the longest of which lasted for 8 years after PTCA, >1 year after PTCA there was not a single recurrence of a lesion successfully treated when the early re-angiogram showed no restenosis. Thus, it may be concluded that successful PTCA changes the vessel morphology in such a way as to make it impossible for the atherosclerotic process to evolve any further.

Among the 87 patients followed up with angiography over an extended period of time, however, 44% developed significant stenoses in other vessel segments and of these 50% could again be treated successfully with PTCA.

The data presented in the paper do not permit a reliable calculation of the risk of patients developing new haemodynamically significant stenoses since the study involving 87 patients focused mainly on recurrence of symptoms (75% of patients). However, within the group of 22 patients that remained asymptomatic, 10 also had new stenoses. Thus, it might be estimated that the risk of haemodynamically insignificant lesions becoming significant, or the risk of developing a completely new stenosis, is approximately 7% per year.

References

1. Anderson HV, Roubin GS, Leimgruber PP, Douglas JS Jr, King SB III, Gruentzig AR. Primary angiographic success rates of percutaneous transluminal coronary angioplasty. Am J Cardiol 1985; 56: 712–71

2. Blackshear JL, O'Callaghan WG, Califf RM. Medical approaches to prevention of restenosis after coronary angioplasty. J Am Coll Cardiol 1987; 9: 834–48

3. Feit A, Reddy CVR, Khan R, Meilman H, El-Sherif N. Changed learning curve for percutaneous transluminal coronary angioplasty. Implication for the future treatment of coronary artery disease. Am J Med 1985; 78: 438–42

4. de Feyter PJ, Serruys PW, van den Brand M et al. Emergency coronary angioplasty in refractory unstable angina. N Engl J Med 1985; 313: 342

5. Holmes DR, Vlietstra RE, Smith HC et al. Restenosis after percutaneous transluminal coronary angioplasty (PTCA): a report from the PTCA Registry of the National Heart, Lung and Blood Institute. Am J Cardiol 1984; 53: 77C–81C

6. Kaltenbach M, Kober G, Scherer D. Mechanische Dilation von Koronararterienstenosen (Transluminale Angioplastie). Z Kardiol 1980; 69: 1–10

7. Kaltenbach M, Kober G, Scherer D, Vallbracht C. Recurrence rate after successful coronary angioplasty. Eur Heart J 1985; 6: 276–81

8. Kober G, Kaltenbach M, Scherer K-D. Möglichkeiten und Grenzen der mechanischen Dilatation von Koronararterienstenosen. Klinikarzt 1980; 9: 869–78

9. Kober G, Scherer D, Koch R, Dowinsky S, Kaltenbach M. Criteria for primary success and longterm results. Analysis of 152 consecutive transluminal coronary angioplasties. In: Kaltenbach M, Grüntzig A, Rentrop K, Bussmann W-D eds. Transluminal coronary angioplasty and intracoronary thrombolysis. Berlin: Springer Verlag 1982: 95–101

10. Kober G, Vallbracht C, Lang H et al. Transluminale koronare Angioplastik 1977–1985. Erfahrungen bei 1000 Eingriffen. Radiologie 1985; 25: 346–53

11. Leimgruber PP, Roubin GS, Hollman J et al. Restenosis after successful coronary angioplasty in patients with single-vessel disease. Circulation 1986; 73: 710

12. Mock MB, Holmes DR Jr, Vlietstra RE et al. Percutaneous transluminal coronary angioplasty (PTCA) in the elderly patient: experience in the National Heart, Lung and Blood Institute PTCA Registry. Am J Cardiol 1984; 53: 89–91C

13. Rapold HJ, David PR, Guiteras Val P, Mata AL, Crean PA, Bourassa MG. Restenosis and its determinants in first and repeat coronary angioplasty. Eur Heart J 1987; 8: 575–86

14. Serruys PW, Luijten HE, Beatt KJ et al. Incidence of restenosis after successful coronary angioplasty: a time-related phenomenon. A quantitative angiographic study in 342 consecutive patients at 1, 2, 3 and 4 months. Circulation 1988; 77: 361–71

15. Thornton MA, Gruentzig AR, Hollman J, King SB III, Douglas JS. Coumadin and aspirin in the prevention of recurrence after transluminal coronary angioplasty: A randomized study. Circulation 1984; 69: 721

16. Vallbracht C, Klepzig H Jr, Giesecke A, Kaltenbach M, Kober G. Transluminale koronare Angioplastik: Parameter eines erhöhten Rezidivrisikos. Z Kardiol 1987; 76: 727–32

17. Vallbracht C, Amuser M, Kober G, Kaltenbach M. How to define restenosis after successful coronary angioplasty. Eur Heart J 1988; 9: Suppl 1, 219 (abstr)

Mehrfachrezidive nach Ballondilatation – Dilatieren oder operieren?

C. Vallbracht, G. Kober, B. Kunkel, R. Hopf, H. Sievert und M. Kaltenbach

Recurrent restenosis after successful transluminal coronary angioplasty – Dilatation or surgery?

Summary: In a total of 333 patients who had undergone a first successful transluminal coronary angioplasty (TCA) of a single stenosis in a native coronary vessel, restenosis occurred in 15% (follow-up angiography was performed in 94% of these patients). The restenosis rate was higher in bypass stenoses (45%) and in reopened vessels (54%). Repeat dilatation of restenoses showed a high primary success rate (93%) and only a few complications (2%). In this group, recurrent restenosis was observed in 33% of patients.

Thirteen patients with recurrent restenoses (11 patients with two recidivations and two patients with three) underwent a total of 41 dilatation attempts. The degree of the recurrent stenoses (prior to the first TCA: 89%; prior to the second: 82%; prior to the third: 74%), the number of eccentric stenoses (8; 7; 5, respectively) and the length of the stenotic obstruction (5.2 mm; 4.7 mm; 4.3 mm, respectively) decreased. Accordingly, exercise tolerance was improved (99 W, 133 W, 146 W). To date, follow-up angiography and functional investigations have been performed in 11 out of 13 patients. Good long-term results have been observed in eight patients and another restenosis in three.

It is concluded that repeat angioplasty is a reasonable therapeutic approach also in patients with recurrent restenosis.

Zusammenfassung: Unter 333 Patienten betrug die Rezidivrate nach Erstdilatation einer Einzelstenose in einem nativen Koronargefäß 15% (Nachangiographierate 94%). Höhere Rezidivraten fanden sich für Bypass-Stenosen (45%) und wiedereröffnete Gefäße (54%). Rezidive waren mit hoher Akuterfolgs- (93%) und niedriger Komplikationsrate (2%) erneut dilatierbar; in dieser Gruppe betrug die Rezidivrate 33%.

Bei 13 Patienten mit Mehrfachrezidiven (11 mit Zweifach- und 2 mit Dreifachrezidiven) erfolgten insgesamt 41 Dilatationen.

Vor dem zweiten und dritten Eingriff zeigte sich ein leichter Rückgang des Stenosegrades im Vergleich zur Erststenose (von $\overline{X}$ = 89% auf $\overline{X}$ = 74%). Der Anteil exzentrischer Stenosen ging von 8 auf 5, die Stenosenlänge von $\overline{X}$ = 5.2 mm auf $\overline{X}$ = 4.3 mm zurück. Die Belastbarkeit war vor der dritten Dilatation höher als vor der ersten. 11 von 13 Patienten wurden bisher angiographisch und funktionell im Mittel 4 Monate nach der letzten Dilatation erneut kontrolliert. Dabei zeigte sich ein gutes Langzeitergebnis bei 8 Patienten. 3 Patienten wiesen ein erneutes Rezidiv auf.

Es wird gefolgert, daß auch bei Mehrfachrezidiven nach Koronardilatation erneute Angioplastien sinnvoll sind.

Einleitung

Neun Jahre nach Durchführung der ersten transluminalen Angioplastik durch Andreas Grüntzig [3] berichten große Zentren weltweit über vergleichbare Akuterfolgsraten zwischen 85 und 90% und Komplikationsraten mit notfallmäßiger Bypass-Operation zwischen 3 und 7% [2]. Ein ungelöstes Hauptproblem stellen dagegen die Rezidive dar.

Von den meisten Autoren werden Rezidivraten um 30% angegeben; auch in der Statistik des NHLBI wurden bei Kontrollangiographien von 557 Patienten im Mittel 6,5 Monate nach Dilatation in 33,6% Rezidive gefunden [4]. Bei Zugrundelegung der gleichen, rein angiographischen Definition (d.h. Verlust von mindestens der Hälfte des ursprünglichen Gewinns oder Wiederzunahme um mindestens 30% im Vergleich zur Situation unmittelbar nach dem Eingriff) konnten wir bei Kontrollangiographien von 333 Patienten im Mittel 5,6 Monate nach dem Eingriff nur eine Rezidivrate von 17% nachweisen [5] (vgl. Tab. 1).

Bei differenzierter Betrachtung ergaben sich deutliche Unterschiede der einzelnen Gruppen; am niedrigsten lag die Rezidivrate nach Erstdilatation von Kranzgefäßstenosen mit 15%. Neben den bekannt hohen Rezidivzahlen von Bypass-Stenosen [1, 5] und wiedereröffneten Verschlüssen [7] zeigten auch die erneut dilatierten Stenosen [5, 11] eine erhöhte Rückfallrate (vgl. Tab. 2).

Tabelle 1. Vergleich der Rezidivraten

Patientengut	Anzahl der kontrollangiographierten Patienten	Zeit nach TCA (Mittelwert in Monaten)	Rezidivrate (%)
NHLBI	557	6,5	33,6
Frankfurt	333	5,6	17

Sonderdruck aus Z Kardiol 76: 428–432, 1987, Springer Berlin Heidelberg

Tabelle 2. Gesamtrezidivrate nach Koronardilatation in Frankfurt: 17 %

Stenosen in nativen Kranzgefäßen	15 %
Bypass-Stenosen	45 %
Rezidivstenosen	33 %
Wiedereröffnete Verschlüsse	54 %

Tabelle 3. Mehrfachrezidive nach Koronardilatation

n = 13, 12 Männer, 1 Frau	
Lokalisation der Stenose	RIA 8
	RCA 4
	RCX 1
Mehrgefäßkrankheit	4
Raucher	11
Übergewicht	6
Hypertonie	2
Diabetes mellitus	2
Hypercholesterinämie	3

Von den Patienten mit Rezidivstenosen wurden 48% erneut dilatiert; 39% wurden bei bestehender klinischer und funktioneller Besserung konservativ weiterbehandelt, und bei 13% wurde eine Bypass-Operation durchgeführt. Rezidivstenosen waren mit einer hohen Akuterfolgsrate (93%) und niedrigen Komplikationsrate (2% notfallmäßige Bypass-Operationen) erneut dilatierbar.

Im folgenden soll über die Erfahrungen mit wiederholter Angioplastik bei Patienten mit Mehrfachrezidiven berichtet werden.

Patienten und Methode

Bei 13 Patienten mit Mehrfachrezidiven (12 Männer und eine Frau; 11 Patienten mit Zweifach- und 2 Patienten mit Dreifachrezidiv) wurden im Zeitraum von Oktober 1981 bis August 1985 insgesamt 41 Dilatationen durchgeführt. Drei dieser Patienten sind im Kollektiv einer früheren Untersuchung enthalten [5], zehn wurden zwischen 1/83 und 1/85 erstmals dilatiert. Das mittlere Alter der Patienten lag bei 65 Jahren; die Verteilung der Stenoselokalisationen wie auch der anamnestischen Risikofaktoren zeigte keine Unterschiede zum Gesamtpatientenkollektiv [8] (vgl. Tab. 3). Alle Eingriffe waren akut erfolgreich; Komplikationen mit notfallmäßiger Bypass-Operation oder Infarkte traten nicht auf.

Der Stenosegrad wurde von zwei unabhängigen Untersuchern jeweils vor Dilatation aus den Angiographiefilmen in Prozent linearer Durchmesserminderung gemessen. Als Bezugsgröße wurde das Mittel des benachbarten proximalen und distalen unveränderten Gefäßsegmentes herangezogen.

Als Umrechnungsfaktor für die Vergrößerung diente der bekannte Durchmesser des Führungskatheters [12].

Als Länge der Stenose wurde der hochgradige Anteil in mm gemessen (vgl. Schemazeichnung, Abb. 1).

Die Exzentrizität oder Konzentrizität wurde aus zwei Ebenen des Angiographiefilmes bestimmt. Eine exzentrische Stenose wurde angenommen, wenn in mindestens

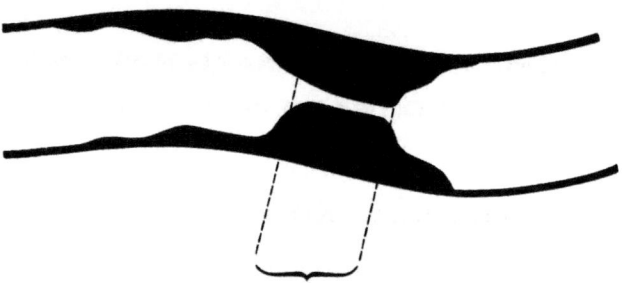

Abb. 1. Schema der Bestimmung der Stenosenlänge (gemessen wird der hochgradige Teil)

einer Ebene das Restlumen auf einer Seite der skizzierten Mittellinie lag [12].

Als funktioneller Parameter wurden ergometrische Belastungsuntersuchungen an der Kletterstufe [6] jeweils vor dem Eingriff ausgewertet und verglichen. Die Belastungshöhe wurde in Watt, die Belastungsdauer in Minuten und der Schweregrad der Angina pectoris in einer Gradierung von 0 bis 3+ festgelegt.

Als Zeitpunkt des Rezidiveintritts wurde annäherungsweise das Wiederauftreten der Angina pectoris angenommen, da bei zuvor bestehender typischer Symptomatik ein Rezidiv in unserem Patientengut in über 80% mit einer wiederaufgetretenen Angina pectoris verbunden war [15]. 11 der 13 Patienten wurden im Mittel 4 Monate nach der letzten [3]. Dilatation angiographisch und funktionell kontrolliert; bei 2 Patienten liegen bisher Kontrollen nur in Form von Belastungsuntersuchungen vor.

Die Definition der Rezidive erfolgte angiographisch nach dem Vorschlag des National Heart, Lung, and Blood Institute [4]:

»Verlust von mindestens der Hälfte des ursprünglichen Gewinns oder Wiederzunahme um mindestens 30% im Vergleich zur Situation unmittelbar nach dem Eingriff.«

Den angiographischen Messungen vor und nach Dilatation und bei den Nachuntersuchungen wurden stets identische Projektionsebenen zugrunde gelegt.

Ergebnisse

Der Stenosegrad im Mittel der 13 Patienten lag vor der ersten Dilatation bei 89%, vor der zweiten Dilatation bei

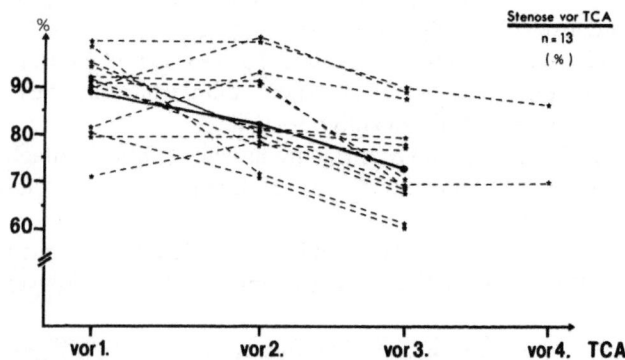

Abb. 2. Stenosegrad in % vor den Eingriffen (Einzelwerte von 13 Patienten)

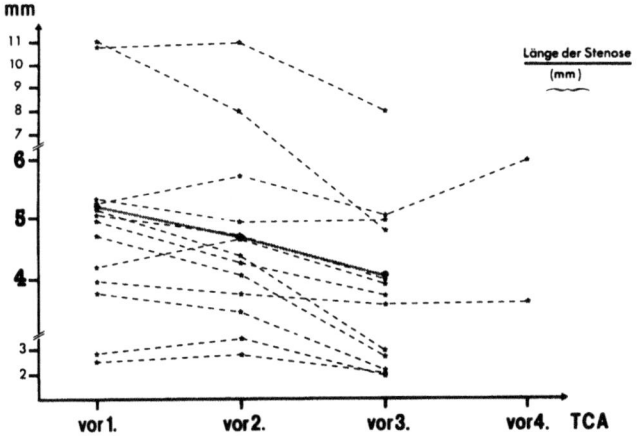

Abb. 3. Stenoselänge in mm vor den Eingriffen (Einzelwerte von 13 Patieten)

Tabelle 4. Kontrollangiographiebefunde 4 Monate nach der dritten Dilatation

Patient Nr.	Erststenose	Kontrolle x̄ 4 Monate nach 3. Dilatation
1	RIA 99 %	80 % → 4. TCA
2	RIA 95 %	steht aus
3	RCA 90 %	20 %
4	RIA 80 %	25 %
5	RIA 95 %	50 %
6	RIA 90 %	80 % → Bypass
7	RIA 80 %	50 %
8	RIA 80 %	30 %
9	RCX 90 %	40 %
10	RCA 80 %	40 %
11	RIA 95 %	50 %
12	RCA 90 %	steht aus
13	RCA 90 %	70 % → 4. TCA

82% und vor der dritten Dilatation bei 74%. In Abbildung 2 sind die Einzelwerte der Patienten dargestellt.

Bei der Messung der Stenosenlänge war ein Rückgang von im Mittel 5,2 mm vor der ersten Dilatation über 4,7 mm vor der zweiten auf 4,3 mm vor der dritten Dilatation festzustellen (Abb. 3 zeigt die Einzelwerte). Der Anteil exzentrischer Stenosen ging von 8 vor der ersten Dilatation über 7 der zweiten auf 5 vor der dritten Dilatation zurück; häufig war eine deutliche Glättung der Konturen erkennbar (Abb. 4).

Die Dauer der Belastbarkeit stieg von im Mittel 3,5 Minuten vor der ersten Dilatation über 4,2 Minuten vor der zweiten auf 5,3 Minuten vor der dritten Dilatation an. Die Höhe der Belastung stieg von im Mittel 98,8 Watt vor der ersten Dilatation über 133 Watt vor der zweiten auf 146,1 Watt vor der dritten Dilatation an, und der Schweregrad der Angina pectoris nahm von im Mittel 1,9 vor der

ersten Dilatation über 1,4 vor der zweiten auf 0,6 vor der dritten Dilatation ab (Abb. 5).

Entsprechend den klinischen Angaben (wiederaufgetretene Angina pectoris) konnte der Eintritt des ersten Rezidivs nach im Mittel 7,7 Wochen, des zweiten Rezidivs nach deutlich längerer Latenz geschätzt werden (11,5 Wochen).

Vier Monate nach der letzten Dilatation wurden bisher 11 der 13 Patienten angiographisch und funktionell kontrolliert.

Dabei zeigte sich bei 8 Patienten ein gutes Langzeitergebnis. Ein Patient wurde bei Mehrgefäßerkrankung und nachgewiesenem drittem Rezidiv Bypass-operiert. Zwei Patienten mit drittem Rezidiv wurden erneut dilatiert (vgl. Tab. 4).

Von diesen ist ein Patient fünf Monate nach der vierten Dilatation beschwerdefrei, bei dem anderen zeigte sich

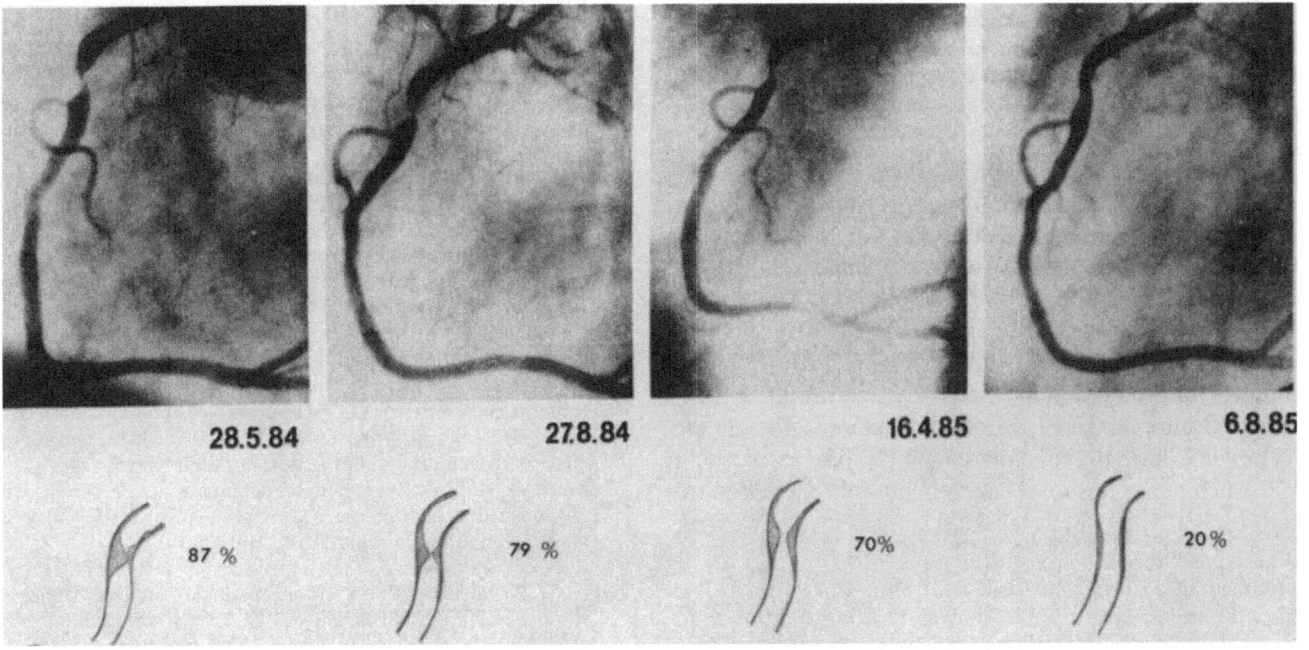

Abb. 4. Proximale Stenose der rechten Kranzarterie mit zweimaligem Rezidiv. Abgebildet ist jeweils die Situation vor der Angioplastik. Das Bild ganz *rechts* zeigt das Langzeitergebnis 4 Monate nach der dritten Dilatation (M. R., 66 Jahre, männlich)

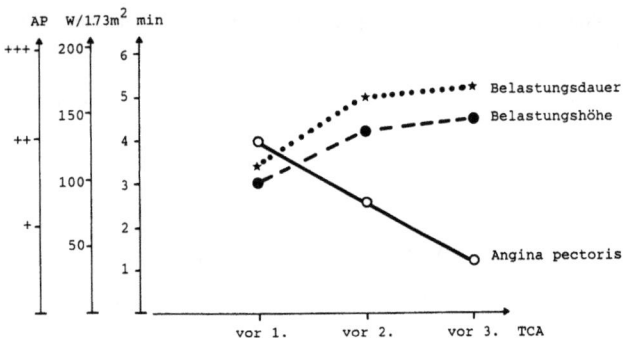

Abb. 5. Belastungs-EKG vor den Eingriffen (Mittelwert von 13 Patienten)

funktionell und angiographisch ein viertes Rezidiv, dessen erneute Dilatation geplant ist.

Diskussion

Rezidive nach erfolgreicher transluminaler Koronarangioplastik treten ganz überwiegend innerhalb der ersten Monate nach dem Eingriff auf [4, 5, 9, 14]; der Häufigkeitsgipfel liegt innerhalb der ersten vier bis acht Wochen. In 80% sind die Rezidive durch das Wiederauftreten einer zuvor bestehenden Angina-pectoris-Symptomatik erkennbar [15].

Rezidivraten sind bei den in der Literatur üblichen rein angiographischen Definitionen [1, 4, 5, 9, 16] nur ausreichend sicher beurteilbar, wenn die Zahl der angiographischen Kontrolluntersuchungen 90% der Patienten übersteigt. Der relativ hohe Anteil der Patienten, die dabei trotz angiographisch definiertem Rezidiv weiter beschwerdefrei oder deutlich gebessert waren und konservativ weiterbehandelt wurden, kann als Hinweis auf die Notwendigkeit einer auch funktionell begründeten Rezidivdefinition gewertet werden.

In den bisherigen Untersuchungen bestehen große Unterschiede in bezug auf die Rezidivhäufigkeit [4, 5, 9]; von den meisten Autoren werden Werte um 30% angegeben.

Diese Unterschiede sind nicht durch unterschiedliche Rezidivdefinitionen erklärbar. Als mögliche Ursachen unserer deutlich niedrigeren Rezidivrate kommen neben unbekannten Faktoren die Auswahl der Patienten, die erfolgreiche Reduktion von Risikofaktoren, die Dilatationstechnik mit möglichst geringer Traumatisierung und insbesondere die konsequente medikamentöse Behandlung vor, während und nach dem Eingriff mit 1,5 g Acetylsalicylsäure, 100 mg Isosorbiddinitrat und 240–480 mg Verapamil bzw. 100 mg Gallopamil pro Tag in Betracht [5]. Auch der in unserem Patientengut sehr niedrige Anteil von Patienten mit instabiler Angina pectoris (weniger als 2%) könnte eine Rolle spielen [13].

Die erneute Dilatation von Rezidivstenosen wird bei hoher Akuterfolgsrate und niedriger Komplikationsrate heute von vielen Autoren als Therapie der Wahl angegeben [10, 11, 16]. Das Risiko dieser Patienten, wieder ein Rezidiv zu entwickeln, erscheint gegenüber der Erstdilatation erhöht [5, 11].

Der Zeitraum bis zum Wiederauftreten der Angina pectoris war bei den hier untersuchten 13 Patienten mit Mehrfachrezidiven beim zweiten Rezidiv deutlich länger als beim ersten. Bei zuvor bestehender typischer Symptomatik erscheint dies ein besserer Parameter zur Einschätzung des Rezidivzeitpunktes als das Datum der angiographischen Kontrolle, das durch unterschiedliche, auch organisatorischen Faktoren beeinflußt werden kann.

In den angiographischen Kontrollen war ein langsamer kontinuierlicher Rückgang des Stenoseausmaßes und der Stenoselänge zu erkennen. Die Konturen der Stenosen wurden zunehmend glatter, der Anteil exzentrischer Einengungen ging zurück.

Funktionell entsprach diesen Befunden die zunehmende Belastungshöhe und Belastungsdauer sowie der Rückgang der Angina pectoris im Belastungs-EKG vor erneuter Dilatation.

Mehrfachrezidive scheinen nach unseren Ergebnissen durch zunehmend bessere morphologische Voraussetzungen für eine erfolgreiche Angioplastik und gegenüber der Erststenose geringere hämodynamische Wirksamkeit gekennzeichnet zu sein.

Die angiographisch und funktionell dokumentierten Langzeitergebnisse bestätigen, daß auch bei Mehrfachrezidiven die wiederholte Koronarangioplastik sinnvoll sein und die bisher in diesen Fällen auch bei Eingefäßerkrankungen häufig durchgeführten Bypass-Operationen meist ersetzen kann.

Literatur

1. Block PC, Cowley MJ, Kaltenbach M, Kent KM, Simpson J (1984) Percutaneous angioplasty of stenosis of bypass graft or of bypass graft anastomotic sites. Am J Cardiol 53: 666–668
2. Bredlau CE, Roubin GS, Leimgruber PP, Douglas JS, King SB III, Grüntzig AR (1985) In hospital morbidity and mortality in patients undergoing elective coronary angioplasty. Circulation 72: 1044–1052
3. Grüntzig A, Myler R, Hanna E, Turina M (1977) Transluminal angioplasty of coronary artery stenoses. Circulation 84: 56–66 (Suppl)
4. Holmes DR, Vlietstra RE, Smith HC, Ventrovec GW, Kent KM, Cowley MJ, Faxon DP, Grüntzig AR, Kelsey SF, Detre KM, van Raden MJ, Mock MB (1984) Restenosis after percutaneous transluminal coronary angioplasty (PTCA): A report from the PTCA registry of the National Heart, Lung, and Blood Institute. Am J Cardiol 53: 77c
5. Kaltenbach M, Kober G, Scherer D, Vallbracht C (1985) Recurrence rate after successful coronary angioplasty. Eur Heart J 6: 276–281
6. Kaltenbach M, Klepzig H, Tschirdewahn M (1964) Die Kletterstufe, eine einfache Vorrichtung für exakt meßbare und reproduzierbare Belastungsuntersuchungen. Med Klin 59: 248
7. Kober G, Hopf R, Reinemer H, Kaltenbach M (1985) Langzeitergebnisse der transluminalen koronaren Angioplastik von chronischen Herzkranzverschlüssen. Z Kardiol 74: 301
8. Kober G, Vallbracht C, Lang H, Bussmann WD, Hopf R, Kunkel B, Kaltenbach M (1985) Transluminale koronare Angioplastik 1977–1985. Erfahrungen bei 1000 Eingriffen. Radiologe 25: 346–353
9. Leimgruber PP, Roubin GS, Hollman J, Cotsonis GA, Meier B, Douglas JS, King SB III, Grüntzig AR (1986) Restenosis after successful coronary angioplasty in patients with single vessel disease. Circulation 73, No 4, 710–717

Sonderdruck aus Z Kardiol 76: 428–432, 1987. Springer Berlin Heidelberg

10. Meier B (1985) Redilatation von Koronarstenosen. Herz 10: 321–326
11. Meier B, King SB III, Grüntzig AR, Douglas JS, Hollman J, Ischinger T, Galan K, Tankersley R (1984) Repeat coronary angioplasty. J Am Coll Cardiol 4: 463–466
12. Meier B, Grüntzig AR, Hollman J, Ischinger T, Bradford JM (1983) Does length or eccentricity of coronary stenoses influence the outcome of transluminal dilatation? Circulation 67: 497–499 (1983)
13. Meyer J, Schmitz H, Erbel R, Böcker-Josephs B, Grenner H, Krebs W, Merx W, Bardos P, Messmer BJ, Minale C, Effert S (1982) Transluminal angioplasty in patients with unstable angina pectoris. In: Kaltenbach M et al (eds): Transluminae coronary angioplasty and intracoronary thrombolysis. Springer-Verlag, Berlin Heidelberg New York, pp 367–371
14. Mock MB, Kent KM, Bentivoglio LG, Block PC, Bourassa M, Cowley MJ, Detre KM, Dorros G, Gosselin J, Grüntzig A, Myler R, Simpson J, Stertzer SH, Williams DO, Mullin SM, Costa B, Mitchell H, and Participating Medical Centers (1982) The National Heart, Lung, and Blood Institute percutaneous transluminal coronary angioplasty registry: The first 1116 cases. In: Kaltenbach M et al (eds) Transluminal coronary angioplasty and intracoronary thrombolysis. Springer-Verlag, Berlin Heidelberg New York, pp 11–19
15. Vallbracht C, Giesecke A, Kaltenbach M, Kober G (1985) Zur Vorhersagbarkeit von Rezidiven nach transluminaler koronarer Angioplastie. Z Kardiol 74: 174 (abstr)
16. Williams DO, Grüntzig AR, Kent KM, Detre KM, Kelsey SF, To T (1984) Efficacy or repeat percutaneous transluminal coronary angioplasty for coronary restenosis. Am J Cardiol 53: 32C–35C

Eingegangen 6. Oktober 1986
akzeptiert 21. April 1987

Für die Verfasser:
Dr. med. C. Vallbracht, Abteilung für Kardiologie, Zentrum der Inneren Medizin, Universitätsklinikum, Theodor-Stern-Kai 7, 6000 Franfurt/Main 70

Analysis of 100 Emergency Aortocoronary Bypass Operations After Percutaneous Transluminal Coronary Angioplasty: Which Patients are at Risk for Large Infarctions?

H. KLEPZIG JR, G. KOBER, P. SATTER, and M. KALTENBACH

Abstract

Severe vascular complications are an inherent risk of percutaneous transluminal coronary angioplasty (PTCA). The data of the first 100 emergency aortocoronary bypass operations required in the first 2850 interventions (3.5%) were retrospectively analyzed in order to identify factors that determine postoperative infarct size. Large infarctions were assumed if the patient died of cardiogenic shock (n = 12), if postoperative angiography demonstrated a decrease in left ventricular ejection fraction by more than 20% or if R-waves in the ECG decreased by more than 40% and a QRS-score increased by more than 5.

According to these definitions, 29 patients experienced large infarctions, 71 no or only small infarctions. The following factors differentiated the two groups: age (58 vs 53 years, p = 0.008), pre-PTCA exercise work load (88 vs 118 Watt, p = 0.0001), exercise ischemia score (2.7 vs 1.9, p = 0.045), degree of pre-PTCA stenosis (83 vs 86%, p = 0.03), coronary multivessel versus single vessel disease (60 vs 38%, p = 0.02), collaterals to the target vessel (10 vs 34%, p = 0.05), total vascular occlusion during PTCA (76 vs 56%, p = 0.035), and long duration of ischemia after onset of the complication (253 vs 179 min, p = 0.012). The data of patients with large postoperative infarctions who survived ranged between those with no or small infarctions and those who died of cardiogenic shock. Higher age (p = 0.04), reduced exercise tolerance (p = 0.0004), absence of collaterals (p = 0.04), and duration of ischemia until reperfusion (p = 0.001) were independent predictors of large postoperative myocardial infarctions.

It is concluded that when complications occur during PTCA, a specific subgroup of patients, i.e. especially patients with reduced exercise tolerance and no visible collaterals to the target vessel, has an increased risk of developing large postoperative myocardial infarctions. In these patients, immediate surgical support should be available.

Key words: Percutaneous transluminal coronary angioplasty; Emergency aortocoronary bypass operation; Myocardial infarction; Mortality

Introduction

Severe vascular dissection or total occlusion during or immediately after percutaneous transluminal coronary angioplasty (PTCA) occurs in 2 to 17% of all cases [1–5]. However, some patients remain totally asymptomatic and can thus be managed conservatively. Others develop severe myocardial ischemia and even die although aortocoronary bypass operation was carried out on an emergency basis. This retrospective study was performed to identify clinical and angiographic risk factors determining the size of postoperative myocardial infarction in patients who underwent emergency aortocoronary bypass surgery after PTCA.

Methods

Patients

This study is based on 2850 transluminal coronary angioplasties that were carried out at our institution between October 1977 and March 1989. Overall primary success rate was 78%, recurrent stenoses occurred in about 20% [6, 7].

The rate of patients requiring immediate aortocoronary bypass surgery due to acute vascular complications steadily declined despite increasing numbers of older patients and patients with multivessel disease. Between October 1977 and June 1987, average rate was 4.6% (92/2000 procedures); during the following 850 interventions it was 1% (8/850).

In 62 patients, the coronary vessel was completely occluded. In 38 patients, long vascular dissections compromised coronary blood flow and caused subjective symptoms and objective signs of severe myocardial ischemia. Ninety-one of these complications occurred during or immediately after PTCA, while the patient was still in the catheterization laboratory. Nine patients with long vascular dissections developed symptoms 30 to 450 minutes after having returned to the general ward. Emergency operation was scheduled if signs of persistent (> 15 min) severe myocardial ischemia (ST-elevation, ST-depression, severe angina) were apparent and reopening attempts not initiated or unsuccessful.

Baseline data of the first 2850 interventions are compared with those of the 100 patients who had emergency surgery (Table 1).

Table 1. Baseline characteristics of the total group of patients who underwent emergency aortocoronary bypass operation and a subgroup of patients who died during or after emergency operation of cardiogenic shock

	Total Group (n = 2850)	Emergency Operation (n = 100)	p	Post-OP Cardiac Deaths (n = 12)	p
Age (years)	55 ± 9	54 ± 8	ns	61 ± 9	0.001
Male	87%	80%	0.02	58%	0.002
History of myocardial infarction	51%	42%	0.04	58%	ns
Coronary single vessel disease	63%	56%	ns	0%	0.0001
Coronary double vessel disease	26%	36%	ns	67%	0.001
Coronary triple vessel disease	11%	8%	ns	33%	0.007
PTCA of LAD[1]	61%	61%	ns	50%	ns
PTCA of LCX	12%	16%	ns	25%	ns
PTCA of RCA[1]	23%	24%	ns	17%	ns
2-Vessel-PTCA	3%	2%	ns	0%	ns
Left Main / Aortocoronary Bypass	4%	1%	ns	8%	ns

p: significance level, calculated vs total group;
ns: not significant;
[1]: patients with multivessel-PTCA included

Exercise ECG

Prior to PTCA, 89 patients underwent exercise stress testing [8, 9]. The tests were performed with an individually defined maximum work load up to a maximum of 6 minutes. ST-segment depression was quantitated by means of a score that considered the amount of ST-depression (in mm), work load and the duration of the test:

$$\text{Ischemia Score} = \frac{\text{ST-Depression} \cdot 100}{\text{Work Load} \cdot \dfrac{\text{Duration of Test}}{6 \text{ minutes}}}$$

Percutaneous transluminal coronary angioplasty

PTCA was carried out according to international standards that were adopted by the American Heart Association [10]. The intervention was performed by either the brachial (90%) or femoral (10%) route. Until 1983, nonsteerable balloon catheters were used. Subsequently, the long-wire technique was applied in most cases [11]. Intraarterial heparin (200 U/kg) was given before the procedure. During PTCA, heparin was continuously administered through the guiding catheter (2000 U/h). Intracoronary nitroglycerin (0.3 mg) was injected before dilatation and repeat doses were given in most cases after PTCA.

In 4 patients with acute coronary occlusion, intracoronary perfusion catheters could be advanced over the guide wire and were placed in the distal vessel. Arterial blood drawn from a femoral artery line was continuously administered (30 to 100 ml/min) [12]. Intraaortic counterpulsation was started in 7 other patients prior to surgery.

Aortocoronary bypass operation

Urgent aortocoronary bypass operation (within 12 hours) was carried out in the first available operating room. The operating theatre and the catheterization laboratory were in the same building.

Forty-one patients received one aortocoronary venous bypass; 48 patients 2 venous grafts; 9 patients 3 venous grafts and two patients more than 3 grafts. Internal mammary arteries were not used.

Total in-hospital mortality was 0.49% (14/2850 procedures). 12 patients died peri- (n=4) or postoperatively (n=8) of cardiogenic shock. Baseline values of this subgroup of patients are separately presented in Table 1. Two patients died 9 and 40 days after surgery, respectively, of extracardiac complications (one septicemia, one multiorgan failure).

Definitions

The degree of pre-PTCA coronary artery stenosis was visually estimated by two independent cardiologists from at least two planes and expressed as percent linear lumen reduction. Stenoses were defined "distal" if they were located beyond the first diagonal branch (LAD), the first marginal branch (LCX) or the crux (RCA).

Intimal dissection was evident when intimal flaps were visible (double lumen contour) or when the coronary vessel was persistently stained by the contrast medium.

Collaterals were found to be present if any collateral filling of the vessel beyond the lesion to be dilated was observed on the pre-PTCA angiogram.

The total duration of myocardial ischemia was defined as time interval between the onset of the vascular complication and reperfusion by the aortocoronary bypass.

Follow-up angiography was proposed to 80 patients. Thirty-eight patients agreed to the investigation. In these patients, judgement of postoperative myocardial infarct size was based on repeat LV angiograms (at 9 ± 3 months). Large myocardial infarctions were assumed if the respective angiograms demonstrated a decrease in global left ventricular ejection fraction by at least 20 absolute percent.

In 50 cases with no postoperative angiograms (48 surviving patients and two postoperative extracardiac deaths), follow-up electrocardiograms (at 20 ± 5 days) were used to determine postoperative infarct size. Two independent ECG parameters were used: an R-wave-score and the QRS-score of Wagner and coworkers [13]. The R-wave-score was calculated as follows: in LAD lesions: sum of R-waves of lead V1 to V6; and in RCA lesions: sum of R-waves of lead II, III, aVF, V5 and V6. Large infarctions were assumed if the sum of R-waves postoperatively decreased by more than 40%. In LCX lesions, the sum of R-waves and the sum of S-waves of lead V1 to V3 were calculated; the percent increase in the R-wave and the percent decrease in the S-wave were averaged; large infarctions were assumed if the change was greater than 40%. In addition to these voltage criteria, an increase in the QRS-score by at least 5 was required to support the diagnosis of a large postoperative myocardial infarction. Finally, large myocardial infarctions were assumed in those patients who postoperatively died of cardiogenic shock (n = 12). In 7 cases, autopsy was performed and the respective clinical diagnosis confirmed.

Group assignment

In order to evaluate risk factors that predispose towards the development of large postoperative myocardial infarctions, patients were divided into two groups. According to the outlined definitions, 71 patients experienced no or only a small myocardial infarction (group 1), 29 patients a large infarction (group 2).

Unequivocal group assignment was possible in 97 of 100 patients (clear-cut anatomical or clinical findings; agreement of angiographic and electrocardiographic findings; agreement of both ECG scores). In 3 of 100 patients in whom angiograms and ECG recordings were available, discrepancies occurred between the two methods. In all these cases, the clinical follow-up and angiographic data permitted clear group assignment.

Data analysis

The following pre-PTCA parameters were analyzed with regard to their influence on postoperative myocardial infarct size: age, sex, history of previous myocardial infarctions, preoperative left ventricular function (ECG-R-wave-score, QRS-score, left ventricular ejection fraction at rest), work load, duration of exercise test, myocardial ischemia during exercise test, percent stenosis of the target vessel, site of the stenosis (proximal or distal), presence of collaterals to the target vessel, number of diseased vessels, type of complication (total occlusion or dissection with reduced blood flow) and duration of myocardial ischemia following onset of complication.

Parametric data were expressed as mean ± standard deviation. Baseline comparisons were made using the unpaired t-test. Frequency comparisons were obtained with either chi-square-statistics or Fisher's exact test. Stepwise linear regression analysis was used to identify independent risk factors for the development of large infarctions.

Variables with significant differences in univariate analysis were included in this analysis. P values of ≤0.05 were considered significant [14].

Results

Baseline data of group 1 patients with no or small postoperative myocardial infarction and group 2 patients with large necrosis are compared in Table 2. Data of group 2 patients were further divided into patients who survived (n = 17) and in those who died (n = 12).

Typical characteristcs of patients with large postoperative infarction in comparison to patients with no or small infarction were: higher age, lower exercise tolerance, more severe myocardial ischemia during exercise, less severe coronary artery stenoses, absence of collaterals, frequent PTCA-related total vascular occlusion, and longer myocardial ischemia (time from the vascular occlusion to reperfusion by the aortocoronary bypass). Only 38% of group 2 patients had coronary single vessel disease, as opposed to 60% of group 1 patients (p = 0.02).

Patients who died peri- or postoperatively of cardiogenic shock showed the most pronounced differences in comparison with group 1 patients (Table 2, last row): 42% of the patients who died were female (only 20% females in the total surgical group); exercise tolerance was markedly lower; age, and the number of diseased vessels were significantly higher; and the duration of myocardial ischemia was significantly longer. Cardiac deaths were only observed in patients with coronary multivessel disease.

The data of patients with large postoperative infarctions who survived ranged between those of group 1 (no or small infarction) and those of the patients who died in group 2: This subgroup showed a trend towards a higher age and a higher percentage of females, exercise tolerance was reduced and duration of myocardial ischemia was more prolonged.

Multivariate analysis revealed that the following parameters independently influenced postoperative infarct size: age (p = 0.04), exercise tolerance (p = 0.0004), duration of exercise test (p = 0.03), collaterals (p = 0.04), and duration of ischemia (p = 0.001).

The frequency of large postoperative infarctions was three times higher in patients without collaterals and with an exercise capacity of less than 100 Watts compared to the remaining patients (46%, 13 of 28 patients, versus 11%, 7 of 61 patients, p < 0.00025).

No final statement could be made regarding the protective effect of intracoronary perfusion catheters or intraaortic counterpulsation because of the small number of patients. Despite the implantation of an intracoronary perfusion device, one of the two patients with low exercise tolerance and no collaterals experienced a large infarction; no infarction occurred, however, in the two remaining cases with a low risk profile. Intraaortic counterpulsation could neither prevent a large infarction in two of three high-risk patients nor in one of 4 low-risk patients.

Table 2. Pre-PTCA data of patients with no or small postoperative myocardial infarction (group 1), patients with large postoperative infarction (group 2), and two subgroups of group 2 (survivors with large infarction and cardiac deaths)

	Group 1 (no/small infarction)		Group 2 (large infarction)			Survivors with Large Infarction (Subgroup of 2)			Cardiac Deaths (Subgroup of 2)		
	n		n		p	n		p	n		p
Age (years)	71	53 ± 8	29	58 ± 9	0.008	17	55 ± 8	ns	12	62 ± 9	0.001
Male		86%		72%	ns		82%	ns		58%	0.012
History of previous myocardial infarction		44%		38%	ns		24%	ns		58%	ns
R-wave-score (mVolt)	70	4.7 ± 2.1	29	5.1 ± 1.9	ns	17	5.0 ± 1.6	ns	12	5.3 ± 2.3	ns
QRS-score	70	0.6 ± 1.6	29	0.3 ± 0.8	ns	17	0.1 ± 0.5	ns	12	0.6 ± 1.1	ns
Left ventricular ejection fraction (%)	63	74 ± 10	26	74 ± 10	ns	16	74 ± 8	ns	10	74 ± 13	ns
Exercise level (Watt)	61	118 ± 28	28	88 ± 38	0.0001	17	95 ± 42	0.02	11	77 ± 28	0.0001
Duration of exercise stress test (s)	61	304 ± 81	28	259 ± 107	0.016	17	286 ± 104	ns	11	215 ± 99	0.001
Ischemia score	61	1.9 ± 2	24	2.7 ± 2.5	0.045	16	2.4 ± 2	ns	8	3.5 ± 3.3	0.023
% Stenosis	71	86 ± 7	29	83 ± 7	0.03	17	84 ± 8	ns	12	82 ± 9	0.044
LAD-PTCA[1]		57%		69%	ns		82%	0.028		50%	ns
LCX-PTCA		16%		14%	ns		6%	ns		25%	ns
RCA-PTCA[1]		26%		17%	ns		17%	ns		16%	ns
Proximal stenosis[1]		89%		90%	ns		100%	ns		75%	ns
Collaterals		34%		10%	0.05		6%	0.012		16%	ns
Number of diseased vessels	71	1.5 ± 0.6	29	1.8 ± 0.7	0.012	17	1.4 ± 0.5	ns	12	2.3 ± 0.5	0.0001
Total vascular occlusions		56%		76%	0.035		82%	0.048		66%	ns
Duration of ischemia	50	179 ± 80	21	253 ± 130	0.012	10	231 ± 87	0.036	11	273 ± 161	0.043

Values are presented as percentage or mean±standard deviation;
[1]: Multivessel-PTCA in two patients;
n: ♯ of observations (for parametric data); p: significance level, calculated vs group 1; ns: not significant

Discussion

Severe coronary vascular complications, an inherent risk of percutaneous transluminal coronary angioplasty, account for the great majority of ischemic complications necessitating emergency aortocoronary bypass surgery [1, 15, 16]. Despite increasing numbers of older patients, patients with previous myocardial infarctions and depressed left ventricular function, and patients with multivessel disease, the total complication rate has not increased in the last decade [4]. The need for emergency aortocoronary bypass operation between 1977 and 1984 (4.8 to 17%) [2, 3, 17, 18] has even declined in the last few years (2.0 to 3.5%) [4, 5, 19, 20]. Results from our hospital confirm this trend. They reflect increases in practical skill, more sophisticated techniques and continuously improving technical equipment.

Several clinical, angiographic and procedural predictors of major PTCA-related complications (death, emergency aortocoronary bypass surgery, myocardial infarction) were recently defined: higher age, female gender, the length of the stenosis, multivessel disease, stenoses at bend points of 45 degrees or more, stenoses at branch points, additional stenoses in the dilated vessel, calcified or eccentric lesions, degree of post-PTCA stenosis, intimal tear or dissection after PTCA [3, 4, 15, 16, 21, 22]. The clinical data of our analysis confirm and extend these findings. In patients with unfavorable postoperative outcome:

- exercise tolerance was reduced,
- fewer collaterals were observed,
- stenoses were less severe,
- PTCA more frequently led to acute total vascular occlusion,
- and the interval between vascular complication and revascularization was longer.

A notable finding of this study was the marked progressive change seen in several variables as one moved from group 1 patients (no or only small infarctions) to the subgroup of group 2 (survivors) to cardiac fatalities of group 2. These variables included: age and exercise-induced myocardial ischemia increased, the percentage of males, degree of stenosis and exercise performance decreased. In accordance with other studies, multivariate analysis confirmed that age was an independent predictor of postoperative infarct size [4]. However, our data also showed that functional parameters are of greater prognostic value than anatomical findings or sex [4, 16, 21]: total work load and duration of exercise stress test, rather than the number of diseased vessels, the site, or the degree of stenosis, reflect more adequately the total myocardial "non-ischemic performance reserve".

The importance of collaterals for the maintenance of myocardial perfusion in severe coronary artery disease is well known. The observation that the presence of collaterals correlates with the severity of coronary obstructions [23–25] may explain our finding that stenoses were less severe in patients with an unfavorable postoperative outcome. Consequently, our data also support observations of Rentrop and coworkers, namely that the clinical outcome of patients after acute vascular occlusion during PTCA is more complicated if the lesion has been less severe [26]. Those patients were obviously less protected by collateral circulation.

Animal experiments [27, 28] and findings in patients with acute myocardial infarctions show that duration of myocardial ischemia [29, 30] highly correlates with the size of evolving myocardial necrosis. Kux and coworkers recently found a close correlation between the duration of myocardial ischemia after PTCA-related vascular complication; the electronmicroscopic results from fresh myocardial biopsy samples; and the postoperative left ventricular function [31]. Irreversible myocardial necrosis and impairment of left ventricular function could only be prevented if the duration of myocardial ischemia (defined in accordance with our protocol as time interval between occurrence of the complication and definitive reperfusion by an aortocoronary bypass) was less than 130 minutes.

Influence of perfusion catheters and intraaortic counterpulsation

Intraaortic counterpulsation and application of perfusion catheters are established methods to reduce the ischemia burden of the myocardium after the onset of vascular complications [3, 12, 32]. The number of patients treated with these techniques in our series was, however, too small to draw conclusions regarding their protective effect. However, our data reveal no evidence that large myocardial infarctions can reliably be prevented by these measures.

Limitation of the study

The retrospective nature of this study led to incomplete data sets in some patients. Informations on exercise testing and duration of myocardial ischemia, in particular,

were not available in all patients. However, the values reported in the result section are most probably valid estimates of the population mean values since no selection bias could be seen in these parameters.

In 50 patients, determination of postoperative infarct size was based on electrocardiographic follow-up. Despite some limitations [33], ECG R-wave-scores [34–36] and the QRS-score [13, 37–40] correlate sufficiently well with infarct size. Moreover, direct comparison of pre-PTCA and postoperative ECG-recordings as done in this study increases reliability of the ECG infarct size estimate. For the following further reasons, the ECG-based group assignment is considered reliable: firstly, because two independent ECG scores were used to determine infarct size. Discrepancies between these two scores were noted only in a few cases and could be resolved. Secondly, because postoperative ECG's were obtained within the first few weeks after surgery when the likelihood of spontaneous reversal of infarct signs is low (one major concern of ECG scores). Thirdly, because we have avoided the difficulty in differentiating between patients without postoperative infarction and patients with only minor postoperative infarction.

Conclusion

The necessity for immediate aortocoronary bypass operation after complication during transluminal coronary angioplasty has substantially declined during the last 11 years. Thus, in low-risk patients, the strategy of using the next available operating theatre for surgical treatment, can be applied. However, more sophisticated measures to reduce ischemia during the time waiting for surgery are to be developed. The presented data characterize a subgroup of high-risk patients with a markedly elevated risk of developing large myocardial infarctions and of dying. These are patients with a large area of myocardium at risk (best characterized by low exercise tolerance (<100 Watt)), and no visible collaterals to the target vessel to be dilated. In these data cases immediate surgical treatment is required.

Acknowledgement: We are indebted to Manfred Skupin, MD, Christoph Kadel, MD, Nicolas Kutzscher and Johannes Schuetz for helping to collect the data and to Brigitte Hallerbach for helping us to prepare the manuscript.

References

1. Dorros G, Cowley MJ, Simpson J, Bentivoglio LG, Block PC, Bourassa M et al. Percutaneous transluminal coronary angioplasty: Report of complications from the National Heart, Lung, and Blood Institute PTCA Registry. Circulation 1983; 67: 723–730

2. Reul GJ, Cooley DA, Hallman GL, Livesay JJ, Frazier OH, Duncan JM et al. Coronary artery bypass for unsuccessful percutaneous transluminal coronary angioplasty. J Thorac Cardiovasc Surg 1984; 88: 685–694

3. Akins CW, Block PC. Surgical intervention for failed percutaneous transluminal coronary angioplasty. Am J Cardiol 1984; 53: 108C–111C

4. Holmes DR Jr, Holubkov R, Vlietstra RE, Kelsey SF, Reeder GS, Dorros G et al. Percutaneous Transluminal Coronary Angioplasty Registry. Comparison of complications during percutaneous transluminal coronary angioplasty from 1977 to 1981 and from 1985 to 1986: The National Heart, Lung, and Blood Institute Percutaneous Transluminal Coronary Angioplasty Registry. J Am Coll Cardiol 1988; 12: 1149–1155

5. Steffenino G, Meier B, Finci L, Velebit V, von Segesser L, Faidutti B et al. Acute complications of elective coronary angioplasty: a review of 500 consecutive procedures. Br Heart J 1988; 59: 151–158

6. Kober G, Vallbracht C, Lang H, Bussmann WD, Hopf R, Kunkel B et al. Transluminale koronare Angioplastik 1977–1985 – Erfahrungen bei 1000 Eingriffen. Radiologe 1985; 25: 346–353

7. Kaltenbach M, Kober G, Scherer D, Vallbracht C. Recurrence rate after successful coronary angioplasty. Eur Heart J 1985; 6: 276–281

8. Kaltenbach M: Exercise testing for cardiac patients. Bern, Stuttgart, Vienna: Hans Huber, 1979

9. Kaltenbach M, Bischofs W, Hopf R, Böhmer D. Physical and physiological work in treadmill testing compared with other types of ergometry. Eur Heart J 1982; 3: 93–99

10. Bourassa MG, Alderman EL, Bertrand M, Fuente L de la, Gratsianski A, Kaltenbach M et al. Report of the joint ISFC/WHO Task Force on coronary angioplasty. Circulation 1988; 78: 780–789

11. Kaltenbach M. The long wire technique – a new technique for steerable balloon catheter dilatation of coronary artery stenoses. Eur Heart J 1984; 5: 1004–1009

12. Hopf R, Kunkel B, Schneider M, Kaltenbach M. Coronary perfusion during transluminal coronary angioplasty (TCA) in acute vascular occlusion. Z Kardiol 1985; 74: 580–584

13. Wagner GS, Freye CJ, Palmeri ST, Roark SF, Stack NC, Ideker RE, Harrell FE Jr, Selvester RH. Evaluation of a QRS scoring system for estimating myocardial infarct size. I. Specificity and observer agreement. Circulation 1982; 65: 342–347

14. Sachs L: Angewandte Statistik. 6th edition. Berlin, Heidelberg, New York, Tokyo: Springer, 1984. 1–552

15. Bredlau CE, Roubin GS, Leimgruber PP, Douglas JS Jr, King III SB, Gruentzig AR. In-hospital morbidity and mortality in patients undergoing elective coronary angioplasty. Circulation 1985; 72: 1044–1052

16. Ellis SG, Roubin GS, King III SB, Douglas JS Jr, Shaw RE, Stertzer SH et al. In-hospital cardiac mortality after acute closure after coronary angioplasty: Analysis of risk factors from 8207 procedures. J Am Coll Cardiol 1988; 11: 211–216

17. Klepzig H Jr, Schraub J, Huber H, Hör G, Kober G, Satter P et al. Aortokoronare Bypass-Operation als Notfalleingriff nach transluminaler koronarer Angioplastik. Welche Faktoren verhindern das Auftreten eines großen Infarktes? Dtsch Med Wschr 1986; 111: 737–741

18. Murphy DA, Craver JM, Jones EL, Gruentzig AR, King III SB, Hatcher CR Jr. Surgical revascularization following unsuccessful percutaneous transluminal coronary angioplasty. J Thorac Cardiovasc Surg 1982; 84: 342–348

19. Simpfendorfer C, Belardi J, Bellamy G, Galan K, Franco I, Hollman J. Frequency, management and follow-up of patients with acute coronary occlusions after percutaneous transluminal coronary angioplasty. Am J Cardiol 1987; 59: 267–269

20. Cowley MJ, Dorros G, Kelsey SF, van Raden M, Detre KM. Acute coronary events associated with percutaneous transluminal coronary angioplasty. Am J Cardiol 1984; 53: 12C–16C

21. Ellis SG, Roubin GS, King III SB, Douglas JS Jr, Weintraub WS, Thomas RG et al. Angiographic and clinical predictors of acute closure after native vessel coronary angioplasty. Circulation 1988; 77: 372–379

22. Ischinger T, Gruentzig AR, Meier B, Galan K. Coronary dissection and total coronary occlusion associated with percutaneous transluminal coronary angioplasty: significance of initial angiographic morphology of coronary stenoses. Circulation 1986; 74: 1371–1378

23. Kober G, Kuck H, Schlinkbäumer M, Kaltenbach M: Vorkommen und Qualität von Kollateralen im Angiogramm bei der koronaren Herzerkrankung. Wertung der Kollateralen mit Hilfe eines Punktesystems (Score). Z Kardiol 1980; 69: 827–834

24. Harris CN, Kaplan MA, Parker DP, Aronow WS, Ellestad MH. Anatomic and functional correlates of intercoronary collateral vessels. Am J Cardiol 1972; 30: 611–614

25. Bartel AG, Behar VS, Peter RH, Orgain ES, Kong Y. Graded exercise stress tests in angiographically documented coronary artery disease. Circulation 1974; 49: 348–356

26. Rentrop KP, Thornton JC, Feit F, van Buskirk M. Determinants and protective potential of coronary arterial collaterals as assessed by an angioplasty model. Am J Cardiol 1988; 61: 677–684

27. Jennings RB, Reimer KA. Factors involved in salvaging ischemic myocardium: effect of reperfusion of arterial blood. Circulation 1983; 68: Suppl I, I-25-36

28. Reimer KA, Lowe JE, Rasmussen MM, Jennings RB. The wavefront phenomenon of ischemic cell death. 1. Myocardial infarct size vs duration of coronary occlusion in dogs. Circulation 1977; 56: 786–794

29. Mathey DG, Sheehan FH, Schofer J, Dodge HT. Time from onset of symptoms to thrombolytic therapy: A major determinant of myocardial salvage in patients with acute transmural infarction. J Am Coll Cardiol 1985; 6: 518–525

30. Gruppo Italiano per lo studio della streptochinasi nell' infarto miocardico (GISSI). Long-term effects of intravenous thrombolysis in acute myocardial infarction: Final report of the GISSI study. Lancet 1987; 8564: 871–874

31. Kux A, Höpp HW, Hombach V, Hannekum A, Arnold G, Hügel W. Global and regional left ventricular function following acute coronary artery occlusion and emergency bypass grafting. Z Kardiol 1988; 77: 165–171

32. Sundram P, Harvey JR, Johnson RG, Schwartz MJ, Baim DS. Benefit of the perfusion catheter for emergency coronary artery grafting after failed percutaneous transluminal coronary angioplasty. Am J Cardiol 1989; 63: 282–285

33. Muller JE, Maroko PR, Braunwald E. Precordial eletrocardiographic mapping – A technique to assess the efficacy of interventions designed to limit infarct size. Circulation 1978; 57: 1–18

34. Hillis LD, Askenazi J, Braunwald E, Radvany P, Muller JE, Fishbein MC et al. Use of changes in the epicardial QRS complex to assess interventions which modify the extent of myocardial necrosis following coronary artery occlusion. Circulation 1976; 54: 591–598

35. Savage RM, Wagner GS, Ideker RE, Podolsky SA, Hackel DB. Correlation of postmortem anatomic findings with electrocardiographic changes in patients with myocardial infarction. Retrospective study of patients with typical anterior and posterior infarcts. Circulation 1977; 55: 279–285

36. v. Essen R, Merx W, Doerr R, Effert S, Silny J, Rau G. QRS mapping in the evaluation of acute anterior myocardial infarction. Circulation 1980; 62: 266–276

37. Handler CE, Ellam SV, Maisey MN, Sowton E. Use of an exercise QRS score and radionuclide left ventricular ejection fraction in assessing prognosis after myocardial infarction. Eur Heart J 1987; 8: 243–253

38. Ideker RE, Wagner GS, Alonso DR, Bishiop SP, Bloor CM, Fallon JT et al. Evaluation of a QRS scoring system for estimating myocardial infarct size. II. Correlation with quantitative anatomic findings for anterior infarcts. Am J Cardiol 1982; 49: 1604–1614

39. Roark SF, Ideker RE, Wagner GS, Alonso DR, Bishop SP, Bloor CM et al. Evaluation of a QRS scoring system for estimating myocardial infarct size. III. Correlation with quantitative anatomic findings for inferior infarcts. Am J Cardiol 1983; 51: 382–389

40. Ward RM, White RD, Ideker RE, Hindman NB, Alonso DR, Bishop SP et al. Evaluation of a QRS scoring system for estimating myocardial infarct size. IV. Correlation with quantitative anatomic findings for posterolateral infarcts. Am J Cardiol 1984; 53: 706–714. In Press in: Eur. Heart J (1991)

Coarctation of the Aorta

Transluminale Angioplastik der Aortenisthmusstenose bei Jugendlichen und Erwachsenen

H. Sievert, W.-D. Bussmann, W. Pfrommer, J. Reuhl und M. Kaltenbach

Bei 11 Patienten im Alter von 5–35 Jahren ($\bar{x} = 25$ Jahre) wurde eine transluminale Angioplastik einer Aortenisthmusstenose durchgeführt; 3 Patienten waren voroperiert. Komplikationen traten nicht auf. Verwendet wurden Ballons mit einem Durchmesser bis zu 20 mm. Bei 2 voroperierten Patienten konnte die Stenose nicht aufgeweitet werden. Bei den anderen 9 Patienten verlief der Eingriff erfolgreich, der Gradient konnte in diesen Fällen von im Mittel 58 ± 17 auf 18 ± 11 mm Hg reduziert werden. Der Durchmesser der Stenose nahm von $4,5 \pm 2,4$ auf $11,9 \pm 5,1$ mm zu. Bei 5 von den bisher 6 nachangiographierten Patienten zeigte sich 3 bzw.12 Monate nach dem Eingriff ein unverändert gutes Ergebnis. Folgerung: Die transluminale Angioplastik der Aortenisthmusstenose kann auch bei Jugendlichen und Erwachsenen mit guten Erfolgsaussichten durchgeführt werden.

Transluminal angioplasty of coarctation of the aorta in juveniles and adults

Percutaneous transluminal ballon angioplasty of coarctation of the aorta was performed on eleven patients, aged 5–35 years (mean 25 years). Three patients had had surgical resection of the coarctation previously. There were no complications. The balloons used had a diameter up to 20 mm and were inflated with pressures of 3–5 bar for 10–60 s. In two of the preoperated patients dilatation was not successful but it was in the remaining nine. In these patients the gradient was reduced from a mean of 58 ± 17 to 18 ± 11 mm Hg, the stenosis diameter being increased from 4.5 ± 2.4 to 11.9 ± 5.1 mm. In five of six patients, angiography three or twelve months postoperatively demonstrated persisting dilatation. It is concluded that this procedure can be successfully used in both juveniles and adults, not only in children.

Die Angioplastik atherosklerotischer Gefäßeinengungen mittels perkutan eingeführter Ballonkatheter ist zu einem bewährten Behandlungsverfahren geworden. Bezüglich der angeborenen Aortenisthmusstenose sind die Erfahrungen noch begrenzt, sie beziehen sich überwiegend auf Kinder mit einer Re- oder Reststenosierung nach operativer Korrektur. Im folgenden berichten wir über Akut- und Langzeitergebnisse bei 11 Jugendlichen und Erwachsenen.

Patienten und Methodik

Es handelte sich um einen weiblichen und 10 männliche Patienten im Alter von 5–35 Jahren, im Mittel von 25 Jahren. In allen Fällen war der Ductus arteriosus Botalli geschlossen, es bestand somit eine Aortenisthmusstenose vom „Erwachsenentyp". Der Druckgradient betrug 30–75 mm Hg, im Mittel 58 mm Hg, der Durchmesser der Stenose 2–11 mm, im Mittel $4,5 \pm 2,4$ mm. In 10 Fällen handelte es sich um eine typische kurzstreckige Stenose (< 15 mm), in einem Fall war die Aorta längerstreckig (40 mm) eingeengt; 6 mal lag eine eher konzentrische, 5 mal eine exzentrische, membranartige Einengung vor. Bei 3 Patienten war 10–20 Jahre zuvor eine operative Korrektur durchgeführt worden; der Gradient betrug bei diesen Patienten jetzt 35, 40 und 70 mm Hg.

Nach Lokalanästhesie und Punktion der rechten A. femoralis wurde die Stenose retrograd mit einem Endlochkatheter oder einem Führungsdraht sondiert. Nach Austausch gegen einen Angiographiekatheter wurde eine Aortographie in posteroanteriorer und seitlicher Projektion durchgeführt. Der Durchmesser der Stenose sowie der Aorta ascendens und descendens wurde unter Anwendung der Verschiebetechnik gemessen bzw. berechnet [7].

Unter Belassen eines Führungsdrahtes wurde der Angiographiekatheter entfernt und der Punktionskanal in der Leiste mit einem 9-F oder 10-F-Dilatator erweitert. Anschließend wurde über den Führungsdraht ein Ballonkatheter eingeführt und bis in die Aortenisthmusstenose vorgeführt. Der Durchmesser des Ballons wurde entsprechend dem prä- bzw. poststenotischen Durchmesser der Aorta gewählt und betrug zwischen 12 und 20 mm. Er wurde mehrfach mit einem Druck von 3–5 bar über jeweils 10–60 s gefüllt, bis die zunächst deutlich sichtbare Einkerbung nicht mehr vorhanden war. Nach Austausch des Ballonkatheters erfolgten erneut eine Druckmessung prä- und poststenotisch und eine Aortographie. Eine Kontrollangiopgraphie wurde 3 Monate (5 Patienten) und (oder) ein Jahr (3 Patienten) nach dem Eingriff durchgeführt.

Ergebnisse

Bei allen Patienten war es möglich, die Aortenisthmusstenose retrograd zu sondieren und einen Ballonkatheter einzuführen. Der prästenotische Druck betrug im Mittel 157 ± 20 mm Hg, der poststenotische Druck 100 ± 21 mm Hg und der systolische Druckgradient 58 ± 17 mm

Hg (Tabelle 1). Der Durchmesser der Stenose betrug im Mittel 4,5 ± 2,4 mm. Es wurden Ballons mit einem Durchmesser von 12–20 mm verwendet. Alle Patienten gaben während der Dilatation einen mehr oder weniger starken, in den Rücken ausstrahlenden Schmerz an.

Bei 2 Patienten, bei denen 10 bzw. 17 Jahre zuvor eine operative Korrektur durchgeführt worden war, kam es beim Versuch, die erkennbar bleibende Einkerbung im Ballon durch hohen Druck zu überwinden, bei einem Druck von 8 bzw. 6 bar zur Ruptur des Ballons. Sie blieb ohne schädliche Folgen, der Ballon ließ sich ohne Schwierigkeiten und vollständig entfernen. Die Stenose und der Gradient blieben unverändert.

Bei den anderen 9 Patienten konnte die Dilatation erfolgreich und ohne Komplikationen durchgeführt werden (Abb. 1). Dabei wurde der Druckgradient von im Mittel 58 ± 17 auf 18 ± 11 mm Hg reduziert. Der Durchmesser der Stenose nahm von 4,5 ± 2,4 auf 11,9 ± 5,1 mm zu. Der nach Riva-Rocci gemessene systolische Blutdruck nahm von im Mittel 150 ± 21 auf 137 ± 13 mm Hg ab ($P < 0,1$). Alle Patienten konnten nach wenigen Tagen aus der stationären Behandlung entlassen werden.

Nach 3 Monaten (5 Patienten) bzw. nach einem Jahr (3 Patienten) hatte der Gradient nur in einem Fall nennenswert zugenommen und betrug im Mittel unverändert 18 mm Hg. Bei einem 5jährigen Jungen fand sich bei der Nachangiographie wieder ein Druckgradient von 33 mm Hg, vergleichbar dem Gradienten vor der Dilatation (30 mm Hg). Unmittelbar nach der Dilatation hatte bei diesem Patienten der Gradient nur 5 mm Hg betragen. Ein Aneurysma hatte sich in keinem Fall entwickelt.

Diskussion

Bei 9 der 11 Patienten konnte die Aortenisthmusstenose erfolgreich dilatiert werden. Der Druckgradient wurde in allen Fällen deutlich reduziert, der Durchmesser der Stenose nahm im Mittel von 4,5 auf 11,9 mm zu. Bei 2 voroperierten Patienten verlief der Eingriff nicht erfolgreich: Vor der Erweiterung der Stenose kam es unter hohem Druck zur Ruptur des Ballons.

Alle Eingriffe verliefen ohne Komplikationen. Die bei 5 Patienten nach 3 Monaten und bei drei Patienten nach einem Jahr durchgeführten Kontrolluntersuchungen zeigten mit der Ausnahme eines 5jährigen Kindes ein unverändert gutes Ergebnis.

Tabelle 1. Druckgradienten vor und nach Dilatation einer Aortenisthmusstenose

Fall	Alter (Jahre), Geschlecht	Zustand nach operativer Korrektur	Gradient (mm Hg)				Besonderheiten
			vor Dilatation	nach Dilatation	nach 3 Monaten	nach 1 Jahr	
1	14 m.		75	35	10	16	
2	25 m.	+	35	18	24	0	
3	25 m.		50	20	–	24	
4	5 m.		30	5	33		Rezidiv
5	19 w.		62	6	0		
6	20 m.	+	56	12			
7	35 m.	+	40	–	32		erfolglos (Ballonruptur)
8	10 m.		70	60			erfolglos (Ballonruptur)
9	29 m.		65	15			
10	26 m.		75	35			
11	26 m.		70	17			

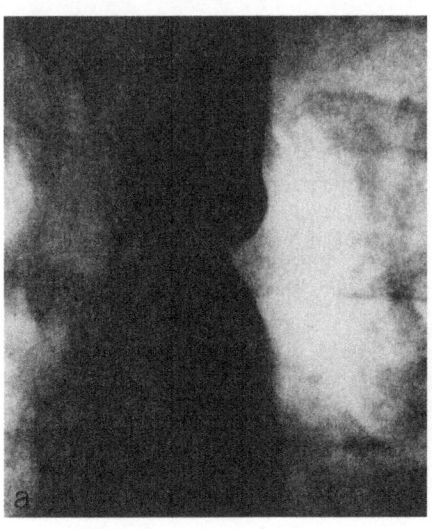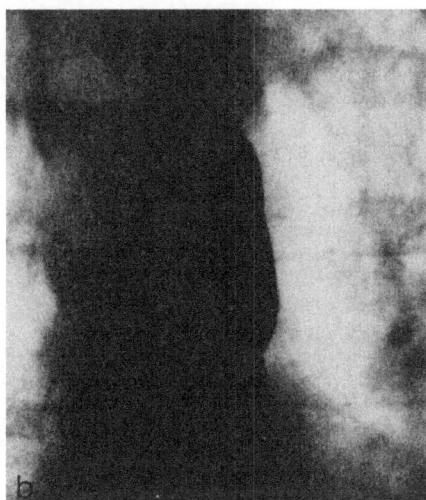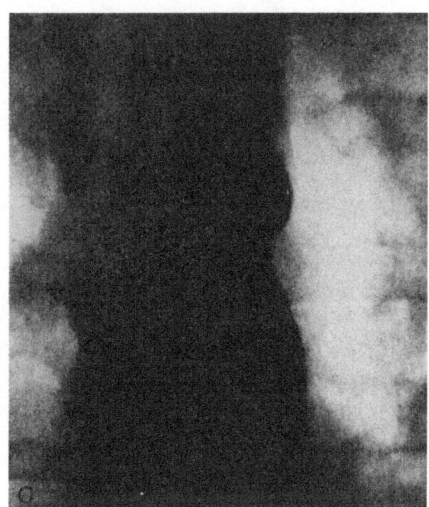

Abb. 1. Aortenisthmusstenose vor (**a**), während (**b**) und nach (**c**) Ballondilatation

Bei atherosklerotischen Gefäßeinengungen kann eine Ballondilatation über eine Kompression der atherosklerotischen Plaques oder deren Volumenverminderung durch Flüssigkeitsabpressung [6] zu einer Erweiterung führen. Demgegenüber erscheint dies bei der angeborenen Aortenisthmusstenose nur durch eine Dissektion von Intima und Media möglich. Das haben sowohl experimentelle Untersuchungen [11] als auch histologische Befunde bei später operierten oder gestorbenen Patienten [5] bestätigt. Bei der Ballondilatation besteht somit grundsätzlich das Risiko einer Aortenruptur. Tatsächlich ist diese Komplikation offenbar selten, bisher wurde sie nur in einem Fall beschrieben [13]. Ein weiterer in der Literatur beschriebener Todesfall ereignete sich beim Versuch, nach erfolgreicher Dilatation der Stenose die Aorta ascendens erneut zu sondieren [5]. Bei versehentlichem Rückzug des Führungsdrahtes nach der Dilatation sollte deshalb auf weitere Druckmessungen oder Kontrastmittelinjektionen proximal der Stenose verzichtet werden.

Nach operativer Korrektur einer Aortenisthmusstenose, aber auch bei nicht voroperierten Patienten bildet sich in etwa 5% ein Aneurysma [4], das u. U. eine Operation bzw. eine Reoperation erforderlich macht. Es ist möglich, daß diese Gefahr auch bei der Ballondilatation besteht. Allerdings wurde bisher eine derartige Komplikation nicht beschrieben. Die Rezidivneigung scheint gering zu sein [3, 9, 10]. Bei bisher 5 nachuntersuchten Patienten sahen wir nur in einem Fall, bei einem 5jährigen Jungen, eine Restenosierung.

Ballondilatationen von Aortenisthmusstenosen wurden bisher überwiegend bei Kindern durchgeführt [1–3, 5, 8–10, 12–14]. Dabei handelte es sich meist um Restenosierungen operativer Korrektur [1, 8–10, 13].

Wie unsere Erfahrungen zeigen, kann dieser Eingriff jedoch offensichtlich auch bei nicht voroperierten Jugendlichen und Erwachsenen mit gutem Erfolg durchgeführt werden. Über Langzeitergebnisse und Komplikationsmöglichkeiten liegen noch nicht genügend Erfahrungen vor. Das Verfahren sollte deshalb in Operationsbereitschaft an Zentren mit einer thoraxchirurgischen Abteilung durchgeführt werden.

Literatur

1. Allen HD, Marx GR, Ovitt TW: Balloon angioplasty for coarctation: Serial evaluation. J Am Coll Cardiol 5 (1985), 405
2. Bussmann W-D, Reifart N, Sievert H, Kaltenbach M: Transfemorale Angioplastik der Aortenisthmusstenose. Dtsch Med Wochenschr 110 (1985), 1839
3. Cooper RS, Ritter SB: Balloon dilatation angioplasty for discrete coarctation of the aorta. Circulation 71, Suppl II (1984), 285
4. Nido PJ del, Williams WG, Coles JG, Moes CAF, Le Blanc J, Hosakawa Y, McLaughlin PR, Trusler GA, Rowe RD, Fowler RS, Izukawa T: Aneurysm formation after patch repair of coarctation. Circulation 72, Suppl III (1985), 47
5. Finley JP, Beaulien RG, Nanton MA, Roy DL: Balloon catheter dilatation of coarctation of the aorta in young infants. Br Heart J 50 (1983), 411
6. Kaltenbach MJ, Beyer J, Walter S, Klepzig H, Schmidts L: Prolonged application of pressure in transluminal coronary angioplasty. Cath Cardiovasc Diagn 10 (1984), 213
7. Kaltenbach M, Schulz W: Kineangiographische Bestimmung von Ventrikelvolumina mit Rechnerhilfe. Dtsch Med Wochenschr 100 (1975), 590
8. Kan JS, White RI, Mitchell SE, Farmlett EJ, Donaboo S, Gardner TJ: Treatment of restenosis of coarctation by percutaneous transluminal angioplasty. Circulation 68 (1983), 1087
9. Lababidi ZA, Daskalopoulos DA, Stoeckle H: Transluminal balloon coarctation angioplasty. Experience whith 27 patients. Am J Cardiol 54 (1984), 1288
10. Lock JE, Bass JL, Amplatz K, Fuhrmann B. WR Castaneda-Zuniga: Balloon dilatation angioplasty of aortic coarctations in infants and children. Circulation 68 (1983), 109
11. Lock JE, Niemi T, Burke BA, Einzig S, Castaneda-Zuniga WR: Transcutaneous angioplasty of experimental aortic coarctation. Circulation 66 (1982), 1280
12. Marvin WJ, Mahoney LT: Balloon angioplasty of unoperated coarctation in young children. J Am Coll Cardiol 5 (1985), 405
13. Soulen RL, Kan J, Mitchel S, White RI: Balloon angioplasty of coarctation restenosis. Evaluation by MRI. Circulation 74, Suppl II (1986), 403
14. Sperling DR, Dorsey TJ, Rowen M, Gazzangia AB: Percutaneous transluminal angiolasty of congenital coarctation of the aorta. Am J Cardiol 51 (1983), 562

Aortenaneurysma nach Dilatation einer Aortenisthmusstenose

H. Sievert, J. Reuhl, R. Schräder, M. Kaltenbach und W.-D. Bussmann

Bei 2 von 23 Patienten, einem 17jährigen Jungen und einer 29jährigen Frau, trat 3 Jahre bzw. ein Jahr nach der Ballondilatation einer Aortenisthmusstenose ein Aneurysma im Dilatationsbereich auf. Der 17jährige Patient war beschwerdefrei, und das Aneurysma war klein (18 mm im Durchmesser), so daß auf eine Operation verzichtet werden konnte und regelmäßige Nachuntersuchungen vorgesehen wurden. Die 29jährige Patientin litt besonders nach körperlicher Belastung zunehmend an Rückenschmerzen. Wegen dieser Beschwerden und der Größe des Aneurysmas (4 cm im Durchmesser) wurde eine Resektion mit Implantation einer Dacronprothese vorgenommen. Der Wert der Ballondilatation einer Aortenisthmusstenose kann noch nicht abschließend beurteilt werden. Alle Patienten sollten nach diesem Eingriff sorgfältig und über längere Zeit nachuntersucht werden.

Aortic aneurysm after balloon dilatation of coarctation of the aorta

An aneurysm in the region of the dilatation occurred in two of 23 patients (a 17-year-old boy and a 29-year-old woman) three and one year, respectively, after balloon dilatation for coarctation of the (thoracic) aorta. The aneurysm in the boy was small (18 mm diameter) and he was symptom-free so that no operation is as yet indicated. But the woman had progressively increasing backache after physical exertion and the aneurysm was 4 cm in diameter. Therefore, the aneurysm and coarcted segment were resected and a Dacron prothesis interposed. As the ultimate value and risk of balloon dilatation of coarctation of the aorta cannot as yet be definitively judged, all patients should be carefully and repeatedly examined over a long period of time.

Seit einigen Jahren ist es technisch möglich, sowohl im Kindesalter [5, 7] als auch bei Erwachsenen [9] eine Aortenisthmusstenose mit einem Ballonkatheter aufzudehnen. Bei der Erweiterung der Stenose kommt es meist zu Intima- und Mediaeinrissen. Deshalb wurden anfangs Aortenrupturen befürchtet. Die Erfahrungen vieler Arbeitsgruppen haben gezeigt, daß dieses Risiko sehr gering ist [1, 7–10]. Offen blieb jedoch, ob sich im Langzeitverlauf Aneurysmen bilden können. Nachuntersuchungen mit einer Nachbeobachtungszeit von 1–3 Jahren zeigten günstige Ergebnisse [9]. Wir haben seit 1985 bei 23 Patienten eine Aortenisthmusstenose dilatiert. Alle Patienten wurden nach 3 Monaten, einem Jahr und 3 Jahren zu Nachuntersuchungen einbestellt. Im folgenden berichten wir über 2 Patienten, bei denen sich ein Jahr bzw. 3 Jahre nach der Dilatation ein Aneurysma gebildet hat.

Kasuistik

Fall 1: Bei dem jetzt 17 Jahre alten Jungen wurde im Alter von 13 Jahren eine Aortenisthmusstenose diagnostiziert. Der Blutdruck war auf 185/80 mm Hg erhöht. An den Beinen wurde ein Druck von 110 mm Hg systolisch gemessen. Über dem Präkordium und am Rücken paravertebral links war ein systolisches Geräusch auskultierbar. Das Elektrokardiogramm zeigte einen Steiltyp. Der Sokolow-Index war mit 6,3 mV oberhalb der Norm. Röntgenologisch wurden Rippenusuren nachgewiesen. Bei der diagnostischen Katheterisierung wurde in der Aorta ascendens ein Druck von 185/110 mm Hg und in der Aorta descendens ein Druck von 115/100 mm Hg gemessen. Der Druckgradient betrug somit 70 mm Hg. Angiographisch zeigte sich ein hochgradig sanduhrförmig eingeengter Aortenisthmus mit einem ausgeprägten Kollateralkreislauf (Abb. 1a).

Im Mai 1985 wurde in Operationsbereitschaft eine Ballondilatation der Aortenisthmusstenose vorgenommen. Der Durchmesser der Aorta proximal und distal der Stenose betrug 16 mm. Es wurde ein 15 mm dicker Ballon verwendet, mit dem die Stenose über etwa 10 s. dilatiert wurde. Die Kontrollangiographie zeigte eine Zunahme des Durchmessers der Stenose von 3 auf 8 mm. Die Gefäßkonturen waren nach der Dilatation jedoch sehr unscharf, was auf einen Einriß der Intima und Media zurückgeführt wurde. Der Druckgradient hatte von 75 auf 35 mm Hg abgenommen (Abb. 1b).

In den folgenden Monaten wurden an den Armen deutlich niedrigere Blutdruckwerte als vor der Dilatation gemessen. Zu einer vollständigen Blutdrucknormalisierung kam es jedoch nicht; 3 Monate später zeigte eine Kontrollangiographie eine Glättung der Gefäßwandkonturen und eine kleine Aussackung nach dorsal (Abb. 1c). Der Durchmesser des Aortenisthmus betrug jetzt 10 mm, der Druckgradient nur noch 10 mm Hg bei einem Druck von 140/100 mm Hg in der Aorta ascendens. Ein Jahr nach der Dilatation wurde eine erneute Aortographie mit Druckmessung durchgeführt, die einen unveränderten Befund ergab. Der Blutdruck an den Armen betrug jetzt im Mittel nur noch 130/80 mm Hg; 3 Jahre nach der Dilatation war der intraaortal gemessene Druckgradient unverändert niedrig. Im Dilatationsbereich hatte jetzt jedoch die umschriebene Aussackung der Aortenwand im

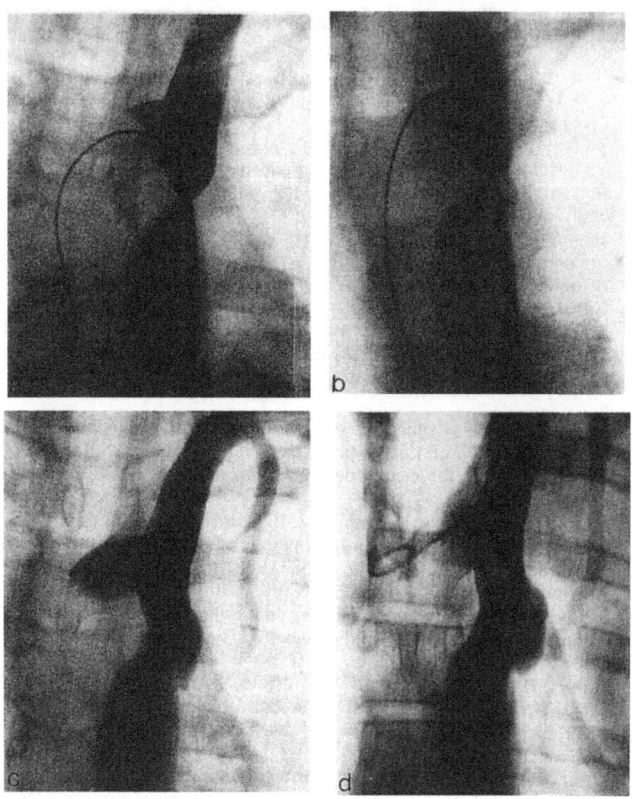

Abb. 1. Dilatation einer hochgradigen Aortenisthmusstenose (**a**) bei einem 14jährigen Jungen. Nach Dilatation zeigt sich eine befriedigende Aufweitung der Stenose (**b**), 3 Monate später eine Glättung der Gefäßwand mit einer umschriebenen Aussackung (**c**). 3 Jahre nach der Dilatation zeigt die Aortographie eine Zunahme dieser Aussackung im Sinne eines kleinen Aneurysmas (**d**)

Sinne eines kleinen Aneurysmas weiter zugenommen (Abb. 1d). Der Durchmesser der Aorta betrug in diesem Bereich jetzt 18 mm und entsprach damit noch dem Durchmesser der Aorta in Höhe des Zwerchfelles. Deshalb und wegen der offenbar nur langsamen Progredienz wurde eine operative Resektion zurückgestellt und wurden regelmäßige Nachuntersuchungen vorgesehen.

Fall 2: Bei der jetzt 29jährigen Patientin wurde im Alter von 19 Jahren eine arterielle Hypertonie und im Alter von 26 Jahren eine Aortenisthmusstenose diagnostiziert. Die Patientin klagte über Belastungsdyspnoe, Kopfschmerzen und eine typische Klaudikation beider Beine nach größeren Wegstrecken. Bei der körperlichen Untersuchung fand sich ein mittellautes systolisches Geräusch links parasternal und ein leises Geräusch links paravertebral. Der Blutdruck an den Armen betrug 150/110 mm Hg. An der A. dorsalis pedis betrug der Druck dopplersonographisch 95 mm Hg systolisch. Die Aortographie zeigte im Bereich des Isthmus eine septumartige hochgradige Einengung (Abb. 2a). Der Druckgradient betrug 50 mm Hg.

Im Juli 1987 wurde eine transluminale Angioplastik vorgenommen. Der Durchmesser der Aorta proximal und distal der Stenose betrug 17 mm. Es wurden 3 Dilatationen mit einem 18-mm-Ballon durchgeführt. Dabei kam es zu einer nahezu vollständigen Entfaltung des Ballons. Während der Dilatation verspürte die Patientin starke

Rückenschmerzen, die innerhalb weniger Minuten abnahmen, jedoch erst nach einigen Stunden ganz verschwanden. Angiographisch zeigte sich eine gute Aufdehnung der Stenose (Abb. 2b). Der Druckgradient hatte auf 20 mm Hg abgenommen. In den folgenden Monaten normalisierte sich der Blutdruck weitgehend (130–140/90 mm Hg). Eine Claudicatio trat nicht mehr auf.

Ein Jahr nach der Dilatation wurde die Patientin nachuntersucht. Sie berichtete über seit einigen Wochen besonders nach körperlicher Anstrengung auftretende Rükkenschmerzen. Der Blutdruck sei normal. Der in der Aorta gemessene Druckgradient betrug 5 mm Hg bei einem Druck von 125/75 mm Hg in der Aorta ascendens. Angiographisch zeigte sich ein 4 cm großes, dorsal gelegenes Aortenaneurysma im dilatierten Bereich (Abb. 2c). Wegen der Größe des Aneurysmas und der Beschwerden der Patientin wurde eine operative Korrektur als indiziert angesehen und umgehend eine Resektion mit Implantation einer Dacronprothese durchgeführt (Prof. Dr. Schlosser, Universität Freiburg). Der Eingriff verlief ohne Komplikationen.

Diskussion

Die Erweiterung einer Aortenisthmusstenose durch eine Ballondilatation ist i. allg. damit verbunden, daß elastische Faserstrukturen in der Gefäßwand zerreißen. Offenbar sind jedoch die noch intakten Schichten der Media und Adventitia in der Lage, dem Aortendruck standzuhalten. im Bereich der zerrissenen Fasern kommt es zu bindegewebiger Narbenheilung. Unklar ist bislang, ob und in welchem Umfang diese Narben auf Dauer dem Aortendruck standhalten. Erste Nachuntersuchungen hatten diesbezüglich günstige Ergebnisse gezeigt [9]. Inzwischen wurden aber von einigen Arbeitsgruppen 1–2 Jahre nch der Dilatétion 10–43% der Patienten Aortenaneurysmen beobachtet [1, 8, 10]. Unsere Befunde decken sich mit diesen Mitteilungen.

Von einigen Autoren wurden auch schon direkt nach der Dilatation erkennbare Erweiterungen der Aorta im Dilatationsbereich als Aneurysma beschrieben [10]. Nach unseren Erfahrungen führt aber der letztlich beabsichtigte Einriß der Gefäßwand immer zu unregelmäßigen Wandkonturen bei der Angiographie ohne Ausbildung eines Aneurysmas im eigentlichen Sinne. Die Häufigkeit von Aneurysmen hängt offensichtlich von der Dauer der Nachbeobachtung ab. Ferner wäre denkbar, daß das Lebensalter von Bedeutung ist. Auch könnte bei Patienten mit einem Rezidiv nach operativer Korrektur infolge starker Vernarbungen die Gefahr eines Aneurysmas geringer sein.

Bei insgesamt 23 Patienten, bei denen die Dilatation einer Aorteninsthmusstenose durchgeführt wurde, fanden wir bei einer Nachbeobachtungszeit von 3 Monaten bis 3 Jahren, im Mittel 13 Monaten, ein großes und ein kleines Aneurysma. Aneurysmen können sich auch im Spontanverlauf bei unbehandelter Aortenisthmusstenose entwickeln und werden auf die mit der Mißbildung häufig einhergehende zystische Medianekrose zurückgeführt. Nach

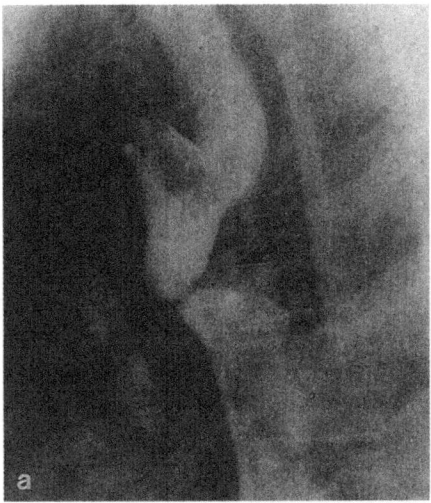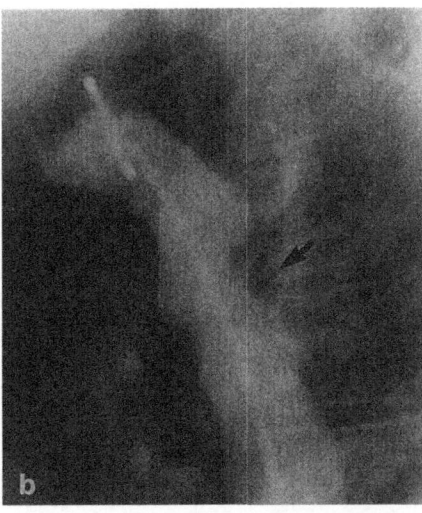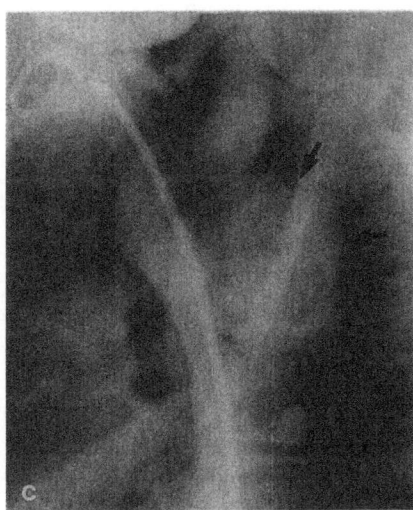

Abb. 2. Dilatation einer Aortenisthmusstenose (a) bei einer 28jährigen Patientin (Fall 2). Direkt nach Dilatation ist die Stenose bis auf 13 mm aufgeweitet (b). Ein Jahr später zeigt sich in diesem Bereich ein 4 cm großes Aneurysma (c)

operativer Korrektur, besonders nach einer Patchplastik, wurden Aneurysmen bei etwa 5 % der Patienten beschrieben [2, 3, 6]. Die Nachbeobachtungszeit war allerdings mit bis zu 30 Jahren erheblich länger.

Aufgrund unserer Beobachtungen halten wir sorgfältige Nachuntersuchungen aller Patienten, bei denen eine Ballondilatation durchgeführt wurde, für erforderlich. Der Stellenwert der Katheterdilatation im Vergleich mit der Operation kann noch nicht abschließend beurteilt werden.

Literatur

1. Cooper RS, Ritter SB, Rothe WB, Chen CK, Griepp R, Golinko RJ: Angioplasty for cocarctation of the aorta. Long-term results. Circulation 75 (1987), 600
2. Nido PJ del, Williams WG, Coles JG, Moes CAF, Le Blanc J, Hosakawa Y, McLaughlin PR, Trusler PA, Rowe RD, Fowler RS, Izukawa T: Aneurysma formation after patch repair of coarctation. Circulation 72, Suppl. III (1985), 47
3. Diekmann M, Hannekum A, Heindel W, Hilger HH: Das Aortenaneurysma als Spätkomplikation nach operativer Korrektur einer Aortenisthmusstenose. Cor Vasa 1 (1987), 255
4. Edwards JE: Aneurysm of the thoracic aorta complicating coarctation. Circulation 48 (1973), 195
5. Finley JP, Beaulien RG, Nanton MA, Roy DL: Balloon catheter dilatation of coarctation of the aorta in young infants. Br Heart J 50 (1983), 411
6. Hehrlein FW, Mulch J, Rautenberg HW, Schlepper M, Scheld HH: Incidence and pathogenesis of late aneurysms after patch graft aortoplasty for coarctation. J Thorac Cardiovasc Surg 92 (1986), 226
7. Lock JE, Bass JL, Amplatz K, Fuhrmann B, Cataneda-Zungia WR: Balloon dilatation angioplasty of aortic coarctations in infants and children. Circulation 68 (1983), 68
8. Morrow WR, Vick GW, Nihill MR, Rokey R, Johnston DL, Hedrick TD, Mullins CE: Balloon dilatation of unoperated coarctation of the aorta. Short- and intermediate-term results. Am J Coll Cardiol 2 (1988), 133
9. Sievert H, Bussmann WD, Pfrommer W, Reuhl J, Kaltenbach M: Transluminale Angioplastik der Aortenisthmusstenose bei Jugendlichen und Erwachsenen. Dtsch Med Wochenschr 112 (1987), 1371
10. Wren C, Peart J, Bain H, Hunter S: Balloon dilatation of unoperated aortic coarctation: immediate results and one year follow up. Br Heart J 58 (1987), 369

Valvuloplasty

Long-term Results of Percutaneous Pulmonary Valvuloplasty in Adults

H. Sievert, G. Kober, W-D. Bussman, J. Reuhl, G. Cieslinski, P. Satter and M. Kaltenbach

We performed percutaneous balloon valvuloplasty of the pulmonary valve in 24 patients (aged 17 to 72 years) and in two juvenile patients. There were no major complications. In almost all the patients the procedure resulted in a successful pressure gradient reduction from a mean of 92 ± 36 mmHg to 43 ± 19 mmHg (P <0.01). In seven patients there was a residual pressure gradient greater than 50 mmHg which, however, decreased in all patients within the following 3–12 months due to a decrease in subvalvular muscular hypertrophy (from a mean of 70 to 35 mmHg). No restenosis was observed. Only one patient, who had calcified valve leaflets, developed pulmonary insufficiency and this was of only minor haemodynamic importance.

Balloon dilatation of the pulmonary valve can be considered a technique with a high success rate and low complication rate even in the elderly. Good long-term results support this approach as the first choice in the treatment of pulmonary valve stenosis.

Introduction

In the fifties, Rubeo-Alvarez and Limon had already attempted to perform pulmonary valvuloplasty using specia catheters [1, 2]. No subsequent reports however were published by this group. In 1979, Semb et al. [3] reported on valvuloplasty using a balloon catheter. Similiar to the Rashkind balloon atrioseptostomy, valvuloplasty was performed by means of inflating a balloon in the pulmonary artery and pulling the balloon into the right ventricle. Three years later the first real percutaneous balloon valvuloplasty was attempted in an 8-year-old child by Kan et al. [4, 5]. Subsequently balloon valvuloplasty has become the method of choice in the treatment of pulmonary stenosis in children [6, 8]. This is a report on the acute and long-term results of percutaneous valvuloplasty in 24 adults and two adolescents.

Patients (Table 1)

Between March 1984 and February 1988 percutaneous balloon valvuloplasty was applied in 26 patients with pulmonary valve stenosis. There were 13 male and 11 female adult patients, whose ages ranged from 17–72 years. The two adolescents were 11 and 15 years old. One female patient had undergone surgical valvuloplasty 20 years before. In three patients the valve leaflets were calcified. Pressure gradients ranged between 48 and 197 mmHg (mean 92 ± 36 mmHg). In seven patients we found a patent foramen ovale. In another patient (No. 23) a pulmonary vein drained into the right atrium. One female patient (No. 15) showed a minor atrial septal defect with a left to right shunt of 30%. There were no other cardiac defects.

Methods

Each patient received heparin i.v. in a dosage of 100 U kg^{-1} before valvuloplasty. Following local anaesthesia the right or left femoral vein was punctured and the pulmonary valve was crossed with an 8F multipurpose catheter or a 7F Swan-Ganz catheter. A pigtail catheter was subsequently inserted into the femoral vein of the other leg and advanced into the right ventricle. After simultaneous measurement of pulmonary artery pressure and right ventricular pressure, a ventriculogram was taken in two projection planes (lateral and posterior-anterior). Video tape recording of the right ventricular angiogram was used to calculate the diameter of the pulmonary annulus.

The pulmonary artery catheter was replaced by a balloon catheter with a diameter equal to that of the pulmonary annulus. In 22 patients we used Meditech balloon catheters with balloon diameters ranging from 18 to 25 mm. In four patients we used trefoil balloon catheters [9]. (Schneider-Medintag) with diameters of 3×10 or 3×12 mm. In the first five consecutive patients balloons were filled with undiluted contrast medium. In the remaining patients the contrast medium was diluted (from 1:4 to 1:10) in order to achieve a faster drainage from the balloon.

The guide wire remained in the right or the left pulmonary artery during dilatation. After dilatation the pressure gradient was again measured. In addition, a ventriculogram was also taken in some patients. After bleeding from the venous puncture site had been stopped by manual compression, we applied a loose compress for several hours. The patients were told to stay in bed until the next morning. After 3 months and again 1 year after valvuloplasty the patients underwent follow-up angiography. In addition, pressure measurements were performed and ventriculograms as well as pulmonary arteriograms were taken.

Key words: Pulmonary stenosis, valvuloplasty, balloon dilatation, pulmonary valvuloplasty

Table 1. Patient characteristics

Patient	Age (years)	Sex	Associated cardiac defects	Peculiarities
1	26	f.	patent foramen ovale	—
2	17	m.	—	—
3	11	f.	patent foramen ovale	—
4	59	m.	—	—
5	56	f.	—	—
6	36	f.	patent foramen ovale	—
7	37	m.	patent foramen ovale	—
8	42	f.	—	—
9	61	m.	patent foramen ovale	—
10	50	m.	—	calcified valve leaflets
11	19	m.	—	—
12	46	m.	—	—
13	21	f.	patent foramen ovale	—
14	49	f.	—	—
15	30	f.	atrial septal defect	—
16	47	f.	—	condition after open valvuloplasty
17	67	m.	patent foramen ovale	calcified valve leaflets
18	17	f.	—	—
19	47	m.	—	—
20	72	m.	—	calcified valve leaflets
21	30	m.	—	—
22	60	m.	—	misleading pulmonary vein
23	46	f.	—	—
24	23	f.	—	—
25	15	m.	—	—
26	31	m.	—	—
$\overline{X}$	39			
s	16			

Results

In all 26 patients we were able to position the balloon in the pulmonary valve orifice. Initially, the inflated balloon always showed a waist which suddenly disappeared with increasing balloon pressure. During dilatation all patients showed frequent ventricular premature beats. One female patient (No. 5) suffered syncope. There were no other complications.

The mean pressure gradient before dilatation was 92 ± 36 mmHg and 43 ± 19 mmHg after dilatation ($P < 0.05$). The extent of gradient reduction differed from patient to patient, but did not depend on the gradient prior to dilatation (Table 2). We tried to choose the balloon diameters according to the size of the pulmonary annulus. Later on, however, measurements from the cine film demonstrated that in individual cases the balloon applied was virtually 25% larger or smaller than the annulus. Within this range, the size of the balloon applied had no effect on the severity of the gradient measured 3 months later (Fig. 1). In seven patients the residual pressure gradient immediately after dilatation was greater than 50 mmHg. On auscultation there were no signs of pulmonary valve incompetence in any of the patients.

The patients had follow-up right heart catheterization after about 3 months ($n = 21$), 1 year ($n = 14$) and 3 years ($n = 3$). In those seven patients who had had gradients exceeding 50 mmHg immediately after percutaneous balloon valvuloplasty, the pressure gradients decreased in five cases after a period of 3 months and in two cases after a period of 1 year, from a mean of 70 mmHg to 38 mmHg ($P < 0.05$). The residual gradient was less than 50 mmHg in all patients (Fig. 2). In none of the patients had the gradient increased to > 50 mmHg (Table 2).

In some cases we could demonstrate that the high residual gradient measured immediately after dilatation was due to subvalvular muscular hypertrophy. Patient No. 12 had a pressure gradient of 130 mmHg before valvuloplasty (Fig. 3a), only 10 mmHg of which were due to subvalvular obstruction. After valvuloplasty the gradient was reduced to 75 mmHg (Fig. 3b). However, 55 mmHg of this gradient were caused by subvalvular obstruction, whereas the real valvular gradient was reduced from 120 to 20 mmHg. This subvalvular muscular obstruction had largely resolved 1 year after valvuloplasty causing a subvalvular gradient of only 13 mmHg. The total gradient had accordingly decreased to 28 mmHg (Fig. 3c).

Auscultation and angiogram of patient No. 17, who had a calcified pulmonary valve, showed pulmonary valve incompetence 3 months after valvuloplasty. Prior to valvuloplasty, his pressure gradient was 85 mmHg; immediately after dilatation, it was 67 mmHg. 3 months later it had further decreased to 35 mmHg. Right ventricular end-diastolic pressure before valvuloplasty was 5 mmHg and 3 months after valvuloplasty 4 mmHg; the pulmonary valve incompetence therefore had no haemodynamic significance.

Reprint from Eur. Heart J. (1989) 10, 712–717, Academic Press, London

Patient	Gradient (mmHg)					Complications
	before	after	3 months later	1 year following	3 years later	
	valvuloplasty					
1	60	25	30	32	25	—
2	143	60	—	30	—	—
3	100	55	38	40	30	—
4	142	83	—	46	49	—
5	61	35	33	—	—	syncope
6	197	30	33	30	—	—
7	48	32	38	23	—	—
8	103	35	38	32	—	—
9	90	30	—	25	—	—
10	115	93	54	30	—	—
11	53	23	38	22	—	—
12	130	75	28	—	—	—
13	88	42	27	—	—	—
14	136	41	15	—	—	—
15	60	25	18	20	—	—
16	54	32	35	35	—	—
17	85	67	35	—	—	pulmonary regurgitation
18	81	56	38	—	—	—
19	75	38	38	32	—	—
20	80	20	17	—	—	—
21	62	32	25	—	—	—
22	70	40	48	—	—	—
23	117	42	28	—	—	—
24	73	37	45	—	—	—
25	105	30	—	—	—	—
26	65	32	—	—	—	—
n	26	26	21	14		
$\overline{X}$	92	43	33	30		
s	± 36	±19	±10	± 7		

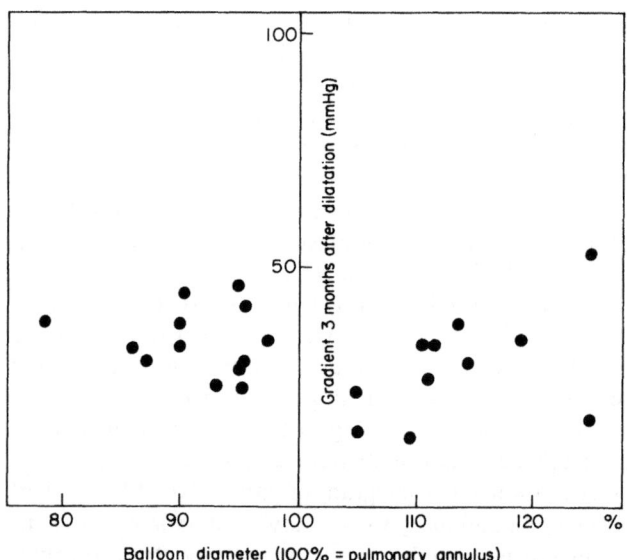

Fig. 1. The pressure gradient 3 months after dilatation did not depend on the balloon size, so long as the balloon diameter was in the range of ± 25% of the diameter of the pulmonary annulus

Discussion

Pulmonary valve stenosis is one of the most common congenital heart diseases. Diagnosis is usually established during childhood and treated when the pressure gradient at rest exceeds 50 mmHg. In recent years surgical valvuloplasty has been largely replaced by percutaneous transluminal balloon valvuloplasty. Only with dysplastic valves, the mobility of which is impaired, surgery cannot be avoided [7].

Percutaneous transluminal balloon valvuloplasty has only been sporadically performed in adults [7, 10–13]. The patients in our study underwent percutaneous balloon valvuloplasty without major complications. One 56-year-old female patient (No. 5) suffered syncope following balloon expansion for a period of about 15 s. Thus, in order to allow a more rapid drainage from the balloon, only diluted contrast medium should be used for balloon inflation. Some authors recommend expansion of the balloon using a manometer for pressure control. This is impractical due to hydrodynamic effects because of the short period of balloon inflation: the manometer does not indicate the pressure within the balloon, but only within the injection syringe. The balloon diameter was chosen according to the size of the pulmonary annulus. However, angiography showed that the balloon had been up to 25% smaller or larger than the annulus in individual patients.

Reprint from Eur. Heart J. (1989) 10, 712–717, Academic Press, London

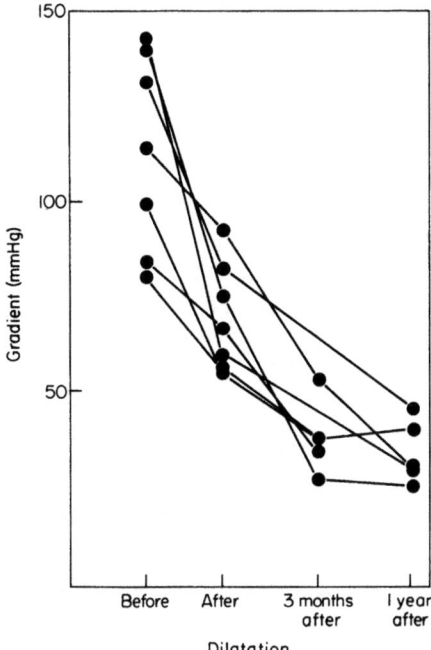

Fig. 2. After dilatation seven patients showed a residual gradient exceeding 50 mmHg. However, in the following months, spontaneous further reduction of pressure gradient was observed.

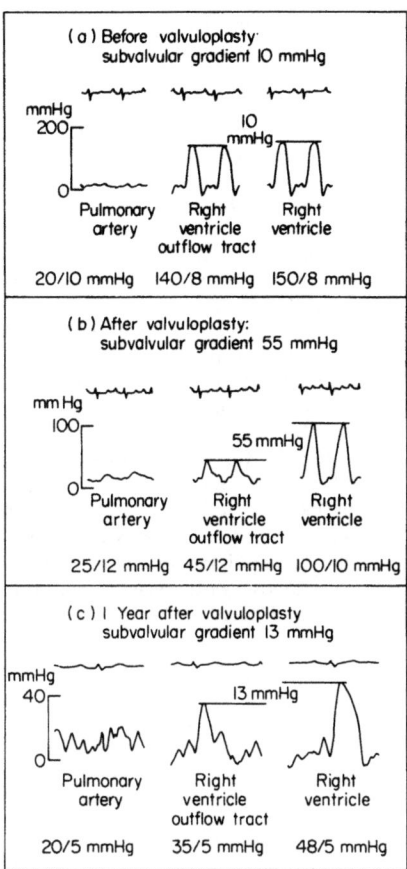

Fig. 3. In isolated cases subvalvular gradients were observed immediately after dilatation (a). These gradients, however, later resolved spontaneously (b, c).

This, however, had no effect on degree of the residual gradient. Since valvuloplasty has been successful and pressure gradients sufficiently reduced in all patients, it does not seem necessary to select a balloon which is larger than the annulus in adults. This, however, may not be valid in children [14].

Percutaneous valvuloplasty can be performed using a double balloon technique [15, 16]. However, since balloon catheters with sufficiently large diameters (25 mmHg, Meditech; 3 × 15 mmHg, Schneider-Medintag) are now available, this technique is not necessary.

In one patient pulmonary valve incompetence was confirmed at the follow-up investigation. However, this defect was of only minor haemodynamic significance. This complication seems to be more frequent after surgical open valvulotomy. It has, however, only minor haemodynamic effects and is usually well tolerated [17].

In our 26 patients the mean pressure gradient of 92 ± 36 mmHg was reduced to a mean of 43 ± 19 mmHg. An observation of great importance in clinical practice is the fact that residual gradients of >50 mmHg can resolve spontaneously [18, 19] after 3 months or even 1 year (patient No. 10). In the subgroup of seven patients with such high residual gradients, the mean pressure gradient decreased from a mean of 70 mmHg to 38 mmHg at follow-up angiography. In isolated cases we were able at the end of the procedure to demonstrate that the high residual gradient was due to subvalvular muscular hypertrophy which spontaneously decreased over several months. Assessing the subvalvular pressure gradient correctly after valvuloplasty, however, is often technically difficult. Thus, this was not achieved in all cases. Comparable findings, however, were made following surgical valvuloplasty [20, 21].

Percutaneous balloon valvuloplasty for the treatment of pulmonary valve stenosis appears to be a safe procedure for adults, showing low complication and high success rates. The long-term results reported here support the value of this procedure and justify this approach as the first choice in the treatment of pulmonary valve stenosis.

References

1. Rubeo-Alvarez V, Limon LR. Treatment of pulmonary valvular stenosis and tricuspid stenosis with a modified cardiac catheter. Proc First National Conference on Cardiovascular Disease, Washington DC, 1950

2. Rubeo-Alvarez V, Limon LR, Soni J. Valvulotomias intracardiacas por medio de un cateter. Arch Inst Cardiol Mexico 1953; 23: 183–92

3. Semb BKH, Tjonneland S, Stake G, Aabyholm G. Balloon valvuloplasty' of congenital pulmonary valve stenosis with tricuspid valve insufficiency. Cardiovasc Radiol 1979; 2: 239–41

4. Kan JS, Anderson J, White RI Jr. Experimental basis for balloon valvuloplasty of congenital pulmonary valvular stenosis. Pediatr Res 1982; 16: 101A

5. Kan JS, White RI, Mitchell SE, Gardner TJ. Percutaneous balloon valvuloplasty: a new method for treating congenital pulmonary valve stenosis. N Engl J Med 1982; 307: 540–2

6. Hagel KJ, Rautenburg HW. Ballondilatation bei angeborenen Pulmonalstenosen im Kindesalter. Herz/Kreislauf 1987; 19: 343–7

Reprint from Eur. Heart J. (1989) 10, 712–717, Academic Press, London

7. Kan JS, White RI, Mitchell SE, Anderson JH, Gardner TJ. Percutaneous transluminal balloon valvuloplasty for pulmonary valve stenosis. Circulation 1984; 69: 554–60

8. Tynan M, Baker EJ, Rohmer J et al. Percutaneous balloon pulmonary valvuloplasty. Br Heart J 1985; 53: 520–4

9. Meier B, Friedli B, Oberhaensli J, Finci L. Trefoil balloon valvuloplasty. Circulation 1986; 74: II-204

10. Bussman W-D, Sievert H, Reifart N. Perkutane Pulmonalklappensprengung. Dtsch med Wschr 1984; 109: 1106–8

11. Bussman W-D, Sievert H, Reifart N, Kober G, Satter P, Kaltenbach M. Perkutane Pulmonalklappensprengung. Z Kardiol 1985; 74: 718–21

12. Lababidi Z, Wu JR. Percutaneous balloon pulmonary valvuloplasty. Am J Cardio 1983; 52: 560–2

13. Pepine CJ, Gessner IH, Feldman RL. Percutaneous balloon valvuloplasty for pulmonic valve stenosis in adults. Am J Cardiol 1982; 50: 1442–5

14. Radtke W, Keane JF, Fellows KE, Lang P, Lock JE. Perkutane Ballon-Dilatation (PBD) der valvulären Pulmonalstenose (PS) mit übergroßen Ballons. Z Kardiol 1986; 75: Suppl 1, 14

15. Khan MAA, Yousef SA, Mullins CE. Percutaneous transluminal balloon pulmonary valvuloplasty for the relief of pulmonary valve stenosis with special reference to double balloon technique. Am Heart J 1986; 109: 158–66

16. Mullins CE, Nihill MR, Vick GW et al. Double balloon technique for dilatation of valvular or vessel stenosis in congenital and acquired heart disease. JACC 1987; 9: 76A

17. Nugent EW, Freedom RM, Nova JJ, Ellison RC, Rowe RD, Nadas AS. Clinical course in pulmonic stenosis. Circulation 1977; 56, Suppl 1, 38

18. Sievert H, Bussmann W-D, Kober G, Pfrommer W, Köhler KP, Kaltenbach M. Ergebnisse der transfemoralen Pulmonalklappensprengung bei Jugendlichen und Erwachsenen. Z Kardiol 1987; 76: Suppl, 1, 44

19. Sievert H, Kober G, Reuhl I, Kaltenbach M, Bussmann W-D. Ergebnisse der Ballonvalvuloplastik bei valvulärer Pulmonalstenose. Herz 1988; 13: 20–3

20. Engle MA, Holswade GR, Goldberg HP, Lukas DS, Glenn F. Regression after open valvotomy of infundibular stenosis accompanying severe pulmonic stenosis. Circulation 1958; 17: 862–73

21. Griffith BP, Hardesty RL, Siewers RD, Lerberg DB, Ferson PF, Bahnson HT. Pulmonary valvulotomy alone for pulmonary stenosis: Results in children with and without muscular infundibular hypertrophy. J. Thorac Cardiovasc Surg 1982; 83: 577–83

Retrograde Mitral Valvuloplasty – A Further Approach to Balloon Commissurotomy

H. SIEVERT, P. KRÄMER, M. KALTENBACH, and G. KOBER

Mitral valve balloon dilatation usually requires transseptal puncture. We performed a mitral valve dilatation without transseptal puncture, introducing guidewires and balloons exclusively from the arterial side in a 37-year-old woman with postrheumatic mitral stenosis. Three months later, pulmonary artery pressure had decreased from 60/35 to 40/20 mmHg and the enddiastolic pressure gradient from 20 to 8 mmHg. The mitral valve area increased from 1.3 to 2. 3 cm². The severely disabled patient was asymptomatic following the procedure. This case demonstrates the possibility of performing retrograde balloon dilatation of the mitral valve without transseptal puncture. (J Interven Cardiol 1989: 2:2)

Introduction

In recent years, percutaneous balloon pulmonary valvuloplasty and aortic valvuloplasty have been adopted for valvular stenosis therapy. There have even been several reports of mitral valvuloplasty [1–8]. However, these mitral valvuloplasty techniques require transseptal puncture. Retrograde catheterization of the mitral valve, on the other hand, is feasible for instance with a Shirey catheter that is advanced via the brachial artery. This report describes a patient in whom mitral valvuloplasty was successfully performed using retrograde catheterization without transseptal puncture.

Postrheumatic mitral stenosis had been confirmed in a female patient many years earlier. Cardiac catheterization was performed at the age of 28. Surgical commissurotomy was recommended, yet refused by the patient. She subsequently complained about serious dyspnea during mild exertion, i.e., ascending one flight of stairs, in spite of sufficient diuretic therapy. On auscultation there was a loud first heart sound and a typical mitral opening snap followed by a diastolic rumble. No rales were audible over the lungs. A chest x ray revealed mitral configuration of the heart and pronounced pulmonary congestion. The electrocardiogram showed sinus rhythm and a P wave enlarged to 0.3 mV and 0.1 sec. The echocardiogram showed the typical clinical picture of mitral stenosis in which the left atrium was enlarged to the size of 5.1 cm. Radionuclide ventriculography showed no signs of mitral regurgitation.

Left and right heart catheterization confirmed marked pulmonary hypertension (60/35 mmHg) as well as an enddiastolic gradient of 20 mmHg between the pulmonary wedge pressure and the pressure in the left ventricle. There was no mitral incompetence. The mitral valve area measured 1.3 cm². Transseptal puncture was not possible for technical reasons.

Therapy and Follow-Up

Percutaneous balloon valvuloplasty was performed without premedication. After puncturing the right femoral artery, a multipurpose catheter was advanced into the left ventricle. 100 U/kg of heparin was administered intravenously. The multipurpose catheter was exchanged for an 8 Fr catheter with a V-shaped tip and positioned as close as possible to the mitral valve. The valve was then crossed retrogradely using a guidewire introduced through the catheter, which was advanced into the left atrium over the guidewire. The wire was then exchanged for a rather stiff, 0.035" guidewire with a soft moulded preformed tip. This wire formed a large loop in the left atrium. Subsequently, a balloon catheter (diameter: 20 mm) was inserted over the guidewire into the mitral valve and inflated several times, but this did not lead to a sufficient reduction in the pressure gradient. Therefore, the 20-mm balloon was withdrawn and exchanged for one measuring 23 mm in diameter. The latter balloon did not show any waist following a single inflation of only a few seconds' duration (Fig. 1).

The procedure was well tolerated by the patient. She did not suffer any disturbance of consciousness nor rhythm disturbances other than mechanically provoked premature ventricular beats during balloon inflation.

Subsequent pressure measurements revealed a drop in pulmonary artery pressure to 30/11 mmHg and a reduction in the gradient across the valve to 10 mmHg. Repeated ventriculography showed that there was no mitral valve incompetence.

Clinically, the patient showed a dramatic improvement of dyspnea on exertion. In everyday life, the patient was completely asymptomatic. At a follow-up investigation 3 months later, after withdrawal of diuretic treatment, the pulmonary pressure measured 40/20 mmHg, the pressure gradient across the mitral valve had decreased to 8 mmHg, and the mitral valve area had increased to 2.3 cm² (Table 1).

Discussion

Transluminal mitral valvuloplasty, which was described initially by Inoue [4], is performed by advancing a balloon catheter transseptally through the left atrium into the

H. Sievert et al.

Reprint from J. of Interventional Cardiology Vol. 2 No. 2, 85–88, 1989
Futura Pub., Mount Kisco

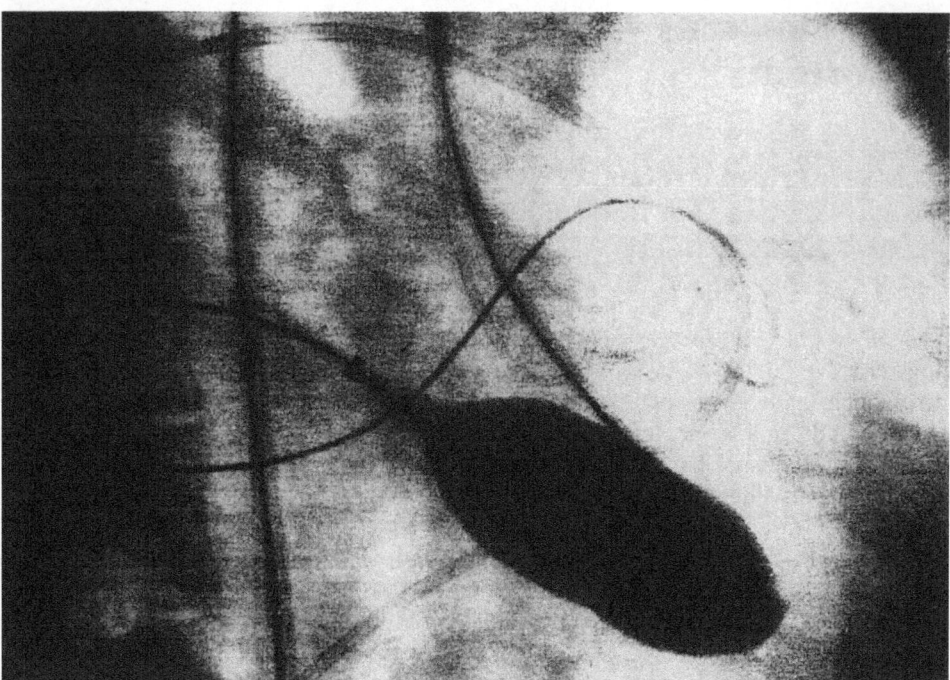

Fig. 1. A 23-mm balloon, inserted from the arterial side, is completely inflated within the mitral valve

Table 1. Pressure Measurements and Calculation of Mitral Valve Area Before and After Valvuloplasty

	Before Valvuloplasty	Valvuloplasty	
		Immediately After Diuretic Therapy	3 Months After
		With	Without
Pulmonary artery pressure (mmHg)	60/35	30/11	40/20
Pulmonary capillary (PC) wedge pressure (mmHg)	30	11	20
Enddiastolic gradient (PC/left ventricle) (mmHg)	20	10	8
Mitral valve area (cm^2)	1.3	–	2.3

mitral valve. It is the technique favoured by most cardiac centers [2-6, 8]. After transseptal puncture, which is associated with several specific risks, the puncture site in the atrial septum has to be dilated for introducing the balloon catheter. The occurrence of an atrial septal defect therefore cannot be ruled out [3]. Babic et al. thus developed a technique for inserting the balloon catheter from the arterial side [1]. In this case, only conventional transseptal puncture is necessary without having to subsequently enlarge the puncture site. After transseptal puncturing, one or two guidewires are advanced into the aorta by means of a Swan-Ganz catheter (Baxter, Puerto Rico). These guidewires are then caught from the arterial side using a snare. The snare catheter is then exchanged for a valvuloplasty catheter. The advantage of this method is that of more easily stabilizing the balloon catheter within the valve and of there being no risk of creating an atrial septal defect. It is precisely for these reasons that we prefer this technique. In the patient described in this article, transseptal puncture was not possible and she refused surgery. We therefore decided to attempt retrograde valvuloplasty.

The advantage of the method described in this report is that neither transseptal puncture nor any catching maneuvre within the aorta are necessary. Provided a suitable guidewire is used, difficulties are encountered in positioning the balloon within the mitral valve. There is a case report in the literature [9] already basically describing this retrograde technique. Büchler and coworkers [9] used a Sones catheter to cross the mitral valve. In our experience this may be rather difficult from the femoral approach. Usually crossing the mitral valve with a guidewire introduced through a preshaped catheter is easier.

The position of retrograde balloon valvuloplasty when compared to the other techniques is, however, still unclear. There might be a higher risk of injuring the chordae tendinae by retrograde crossing of the mitral valve. Moreover, antegrade crossing is easier. Thus, retrograde balloon valvuloplasty of the mitral valve should only be considered when transseptal puncture fails or when it is not

Reprint from J. of Interventional Cardiology Vol. 2 No. 2, 85–88, 1989
Futura Pub., Mount Kisco

possible to advance the balloon catheter through the atrial septum and to position it within the mitral valve.

References

1. Babic UU, Vucinic M, Grujicic SM. Percutaneous transarterial balloon valvuloplasty for end-stage mitral valve stenosis. Scand J Thor Carciovasc Surg 1986; 20: 189–191

2. Bussmann W-D, Sievert H, Reifart N, et al. Transfemorale Valvuloplastik mit dem Ballonkatheter bei Mitralstenose. Dtsch med Wochensch 1987; 112: 842–844

3. Diver DJ, Safian RD, Berman AD, et al. Percutaneous balloon mitral valvuloplasty: Acute results and long term follow-up. J Am Coll Cardiol 1987; 9:14

4. Inoue K, Owaki T, Nakamura T, et al. Clinical application of transvenous mitral commissurotomy by a new balloon catheter. J Thorac Cardiovasc Surg 1984; 87: 394–402

5. Lock JE, Khalilullah M, Shrivastava S, et al. Percutaneous catheter commissurotomy in rheumatic mitral stenosis. N Engl J Med 1985; 313: 1515–1518

6. Palacios J, Block PC, Brandi S, et al. Percutaneous balloon valvotomy for patients with severe mitral stenosis. Circulation 1987; 75: 778–784

7. Sievert H, Kober G, Bussmann W-D, et al. Kathetervalvuloplastik der Mitralstenose. Dtsch Med Wschr 1989; 114: 248–252

8. Al Zaibag M, Ribeiro PA, Al Kasab S, et al. Percutaneous double balloon mitral valvotomy for rheumatic mitral stenosis. Lancet 1986; 1: 757–761

9. Büchler JR, Fo SFA, Braga SLN, et al. Percutaneous mitral valvuloplasty in rheumatic mitral stenosis by isolated transarterial approach. Jpn Heart J 1987; 28: 791–798

Transluminale Valvuloplastik der nicht verkalkten Aortenstenose: Akut- und Langzeitergebnisse

H. Sievert, P. Krämer, W.-D. Bussmann, M. Kaltenbach und G. Kober

Bei 6 Patienten, 2 Frauen und 4 Männern, im Alter von 11–44 Jahren (Mittel: 24 ± 11 Jahre) mit einer nicht verkalkten Aortenklappenstenose wurde der Versuch einer transfemoralen Ballondilatation unternommen. In 5 Fällen konnte ein Ballon in der Klappe plaziert und vollständig gefüllt werden. Bei einer Patientin mißlang der Eingriff wegen damals noch bestehender technischer Probleme. Der Druckgradient wurde von im Mittel 83 ± 26 auf 42 ± 20 mmHg reduziert. Schwere Komplikationen traten nicht auf. Eine bei 3 Patienten vorbestehende geringgradige Aorteninsuffizienz wurde nicht verstärkt, bei den anderen beiden Patienten wurde keine Aorteninsuffizienz erzeugt. Bei der Nachuntersuchung nach 3 Monaten bzw. einem Jahr hatte der Gradient bei zwei Patienten wieder auf 50 bzw. 110 mmHg zugenommen. Ein Patient wurde nochmals dilatiert, der zweite operiert. Unter Berücksichtigung der Spätkomplikationen nach operativem Aortenklappenersatz ist bei nicht verkalkter – anders als bei verkalkter – Aortenstenose der Versuch einer Ballondilatation gerechtfertigt, unter Umständen allein mit dem Ziel, den Zeitpunkt einer eventuell doch noch erforderlichen Operation hinauszuschieben. Langzeitbeobachtungen über viele Jahre müssen zeigen, ob sich in Einzelfällen eine Operation vollständig vermeiden läßt.

Transfemoral percutaneous balloon valvuloplasty was attempted in the case of 6 patients (2 females and 4 males aged 11 to 44 years, mean: 24 ± 11 years) with uncalcified aortic valve stenosis. In 5 patients we were able to cross the valve and inflate the balloon. Due to technical problems at that time, however, the attempt was unsuccessful in one female patient. Pressure gradients were reduced from a mean of 83 ± 26 to 42 ± 20 mmHg. There were no major complications. Pre-existing minor aortic incompetence in 3 patients did not deteriorate and the remaining 2 patients did not develop aortic incompetence. Follow-up investigations performed twice – 3 months and 1 year after valvuloplasty – showed that pressure gradients had increased in two cases to a value of 50 to 110 mmHg, respectively. One of them underwent repeat transfemoral percutaneous balloon valvuloplasty, the other one was operated.

Schlüsselwörter: Aortenstenose, Ballondilatation, transluminale Valvuloplastik
Key words: aortic stenosis, balloon dilatation, transluminal valvuloplasty

Taking into consideration late complications following aortic valve replacement, the attempt of percutaneous balloon valvuloplasty is recommended with uncalcified aortic stenosis, even if the only objective is to postpone surgery. Long-term follow-up investigations will have to prove whether surgery can be avoided in some of the patients.

Die Ballondilatation der Aortenstenose bei Kindern wurde erstmals 1984 von Lababidi et al. [7] beschrieben. Da die Diagnose einer angeborenen Aortenstenose schon wegen des eindrucksvollen Auskultationsbefundes meist bereits im Kindesalter gestellt wird, ist das Krankheitsbild im Erwachsenenalter relativ selten. Hier sind wesentlich häufiger sekundär durch Verkalkung entstandene Aortenstenosen bei angeborenen Fehlbildungen der Aortenklappe (bikuspide Klappe), postrheumatische Vitien und die senile Form der Aortenstenose. Dementsprechend gering sind die Erfahrungen mit der transluminalen Ballondilatation nicht verkalkter Aortenstenosen jenseits des Kindesalters [1, 8, 10, 12].

Im folgenden berichten wir über Akut- und Langzeitergebnisse der transfemoralen Ballondilatation bei 6 Patienten.

Patienten

Von 1984–1988 wurde bei 6 Patienten (4 Männer und 2 Frauen) der Versuch einer transfemoralen Ballondilatation einer angeborenen, nicht verkalkten Aortenstenose unternommen. Der jüngste Patient war 11 Jahre, der älteste 44 Jahre alt. Das Durchschnittsalter betrug 24 ± 11 Jahre. Bei zwei Patienten (Nr. 3 und 4) war im Kleinkindesalter eine Aortenisthmusstenose operativ korrigiert worden. Subjektiv klagten alle Patienten über belastungsabhängige Atemnot. Alle Patienten boten elektrokardiographisch die Zeichen einer Linksherzhypertrophie. Der Sokolow-Index betrug im Mittel 5 ± 1,3 mV. Das röntgenologisch bestimmte Herzvolumen war bei allen Patienten noch normal (obere Normgrenze bei Frauen: 700, bei Männern: 800 ml/1,73 m²) und betrug im Mittel 700 ± 17,4 ml/1,73 m². Der Druckgradient zwischen linkem Ventrikel und der Aorta betrug bei allen Patienten über 50 mmHg (60–130 mmHg) und lag im Mittel bei 83 mmHg. Bei der Aortographie zeigte sich in 3 Fällen (Patienten Nr. 1, 2, 5) ein geringfügiger Kontrastmittelrückfluß in den linken Ventrikel.

Bei einem Patienten (Nr. 4) wurde wegen eines mäßigen Wiederanstiegs des Gradienten nach einem Jahr eine zweite Dilatation durchgeführt.

Methodik

Nach Punktion der rechten oder linken Arteria femoralis wurde unter Antikoagulation mit Heparin (100 E/kg Körpergewicht) die Aortenklappe mit einem Führungsdraht und einem Sones-Katheter sondiert. Nach der Druckregistrierung wurde der Sones-Katheter über einen 260 cm langen Wechseldraht gegen einen Ballonkatheter ausgetauscht. Ab Patient Nr. 5 wurde hierzu ein sehr harter Draht mit weicher, gebogener Spitze verwendet. Bei Patient Nr. 1 wurde der Ballonkatheter durch eine Schleuse, bei allen anderen direkt perkutan eingeführt. Der Durchmesser des Ballons betrug 20 bzw. 23 mm, bei 2 Patienten wurde ein Trifoil-Ballon mit 3 × 12 mm (Patient Nr. 6) bzw. 3 × 10 mm (Patient Nr. 4) Durchmeser verwendet. Die Ballongröße wurde möglichst 1–2 mm kleiner, keinesfalls jedoch größer als dem angiographisch ermittelten Durchmesser des Aortenklappenringes entsprechend gewählt. Der Ballon wurde von Hand über 5–10 s mit 1:5 bis 1:10 verdünntem Kontrastmittel gefüllt. Dabei wurde wegen der Kürze der Füllungszeit, die eine zuverlässige Druckmessung im Ballon nicht ermöglicht, auf ein Manometer verzichtet. Nach der Dilatation erfolgte eine erneute Druckregistrierung und eine Aortographie. Die Blutstillung erfolgte durch manuelle Kompression. Vor und für 24 Std. nach dem Eingriff erfolgte eine Endokarditisprophylaxe. Nach 3 Monaten und/oder einem Jahr wurde eine Nachuntersuchung mit Registrierung der Drücke und Angiokardiographie durchgeführt.

Ergebnisse (Tab. I)

Bei einer Patientin (Nr. 2) mit stark erweiterter und elongierter Aorta ascendens konnte der linke Ventrikel wohl mit einem Führungsdraht, nicht jedoch mit einem Katheter sondiert werden – eine Schwierigkeit, die durch technische Verbesserungen heute vermieden werden kann. Sie wurde später operiert, wobei es notwendig war, die Klappe durch eine Kunstklappe zu ersetzen. In den anderen Fällen konnte ein Ballonkatheter in der Klappe plaziert und gefüllt werden. Im Einzelfall erwies es sich als sehr schwierig, den Ballon während der Insufflation in der Klappe zu stabilisieren. Dies wurde durch die Verwendung härterer Führungsdrähte wesentlich erleichtert. Während der Dilatation traten stets zahlreiche ventrikuläre Extrasystolen auf. Vor der Dilatation betrug der systolische Druckgradient 60–130 mmHg, im Mittel 83 ±

26 mmHg, nach der Dilatation 20–75, im Mittel 42 ± 20 mmHg. Bei einer Patientin verblieb ein Gradient von 75 mmHg, bei den anderen 4 Patienten wurde der Gradient auf weniger als 50 mmHg reduziert. Der bei 3 Patienten bestehende geringfügige Kontrastmittelrückfluß in den linken Ventrikel bei der Aortographie nahm nach Dilatation nicht zu, bei den übrigen 2 Patienten entstand keine angiographisch erkennbare Aorteninsuffizienz.

Alle erfolgreich dilatierten Patienten waren nach dem Eingriff beschwerdefrei. Bei der Nachangiographie nach drei Monaten bzw. einem Jahr betrug der Druckgradient 35, 30, 50, 105 bzw. 25 mmHg. Bei dem Patienten Nr. 4 wurde unter Verwendung eines größeren Ballons (3 × 12 mm) nochmals eine Dilatation durchgeführt. Dadurch konnte der Druckgradient von 50 auf 30 mmHg reduziert werden. Bei der Patientin Nr. 5 wurde ein Aortenklappenersatz durchgeführt. Intraoperativ zeigte sich eine stark verdickte und verwachsene bikuspide Klappe. Eine Kommissur war auf eine Länge von 2 mm eingerissen (Abb. 1). Die Klappe wurde entfernt und durch eine Kunstprothese ersetzt.

Diskussion

Die Ballondilatation der angeborenen Pulmonalstenose ist im Kindesalter ein inzwischen weit verbreitetes etabliertes Verfahren [2, 4]. Auch im Erwachsenenalter wur-

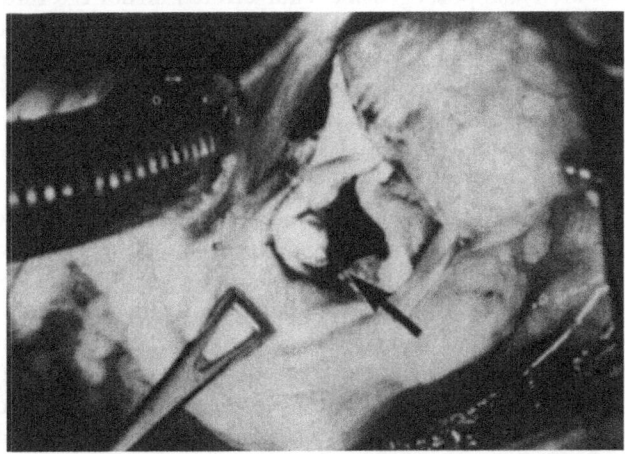

Abb. 1. Bei einer 26jährigen Patientin wurde wegen eines ungenügenden Dilatationserfolgs ein Aortenklappenersatz vorgenommen. Intraoperativ zeigte sich eine stark verdickte bikuspide Klappe mit einem Einriß einer Kommissur (Pfeil)

Tabelle 1. Akut- und Langzeitergebnisse der Ballondilatation bei nicht verkalkter Aortenstenose

Patient	Systolischer Druckgradient		nach 3 Monaten	nach 1 Jahr	Verlauf
	vorher	nachher			
1 (23) m	60	40	35*	35**	
2 (44) w	90	—	—	—	AKE
3 (11) m	80	40	20	30	
4 (16) m	75	35	60	50 → 30***	
5 /26) w	130	75	105	—	AKE
6 (21) m	60	20	25		

* = nach 6 Monaten; ** = nach 3 Jahren; *** = zweite Ballondilatation; AKE = Aortenklappenersatz

den günstige Ergebnisse erzielt [14], die es als Behandlungsmethode der Wahl erscheinen läßt. Ballondilatationen der nicht verkalkten Aortenstenose wurden überwiegend bei Kindern durchgeführt [5–10, 15]. Da mißgebildete Aortenklappen mehr als Pulmonalklappen im Laufe des Lebens zu Fibrosierung und nachfolgend zu Verkalkung neigen, war mit ungünstigeren Ergebnissen bei Erwachsenen zu rechnen. Hinzu kommt, daß der Eingriff durch Elongation und Erweiterung der Aorta sowie das größere Füllvolumen des Ballons technisch schwieriger ist [8, 14]. Bei einem Druckgradienten von über 50 mmHg gilt ein Aortenklappenersatz bzw., wenn technisch möglich, eine operative Valvuloplastik als indiziert. Daran gemessen war der Akuterfolg der Ballondilatation bei 4 der 6 Patienten als zufriedenstellend zu bezeichnen. Bei einer Patientin konnte zwar die Dilatation durchgeführt werden, der Gradient wurde jedoch nicht ausreichend reduziert.

Der Mechanismus der Aortenklappendilatation bei nichtverkalkter Klappe besteht, wie anhand des Falles Nr. 5 demonstriert werden konnte, in einem Einriß einer Kommissur. Daneben ist auch eine Dehnung der Klappensegel möglich. Dies könnte die erneute Zunahme des Gradienten innerhalb kurzer Zeit bei zwei Patienten (Nr. 4 und 5) erklären. Insgesamt sind jedoch die jetzt vorliegenden Langzeitverläufe wesentlich günstiger als bei verkalkten Aortenklappen, bei denen wir eine Ballondilatation nur noch in seltenen Fällen durchführen [13].

Komplikationen sind bei unseren Patienten mit nicht verkalkten Klappensegeln nicht aufgetreten. In der Literatur sind jedoch – meist bei Kindern – Verletzungen und Thrombosen der Arteria femoralis, Nachblutungen, Kammerflimmern, Perikardtamponaden und auch Todesfälle beschrieben [1, 5, 8]. Möglich, nach der Literatur jedoch selten ist die Entstehung einer schweren Aorteninsuffizienz [7].

Das Verfahren ist technisch wesentlich schwieriger als die Dilatation von Pulmonalklappen. Es sollte deshalb nur in spezialisierten Zentren angewandt werden. Grundsätzlich handelt es sich wie auch bei der operativen Valvuloplastik [3, 11] um ein palliatives Verfahren. Langfristig ist nach transluminaler Valvuloplastik eine Verkalkung und hierdurch eine Restenosierung der Klappe vorstellbar, so daß nach Jahren ein Klappenersatz notwendig werden kann. Langzeitbeobachtungen über viele Jahre und Jahrzehnte nach aortaler Valvuloplastik müssen hierüber Aufschluß geben. Unter Berücksichtigung der nicht unbegrenzten Haltbarkeit von Klappenprothesen und der Problematik einer lebenslangen Antikoagulation stellt jedoch der Aufschub der Operation um Jahre einen Gewinn dar. Deshalb sollte vor einem operativen Eingriff eine Ballondilatation erwogen werden.

Literatur

1. Erdmann E, Höfling B: Perkutane transfemorale Valvuloplastie der verkalkten und nicht verkalkten Aortenklappe. DMW 112, 1067 (1987)
2. Hagel KJ, Rautenburg HW: Ballondilatation bei angeborenen Pulmonalstenosen im Kindesalter. Herz/Kreisl. 19, 343 (1987)
3. Hsieh KS, Keane JF, Bernhard WF, Nadas AS, Castaneda AR: Long-term follow-up of children after aortic valvulotomy. Circulation 70 (Suppl. II) 132 (1984)
4. Kan JS, White RI, Mitchell SE, Anderson JH, Gardner TJ: Percutaneous transluminal balloon valvuloplasty for pulmonary stenosis. Circulation 69, 554 (1984)
5. Keane JF, Helgason H, Fellows KE, Lock JE: Results and complications of balloon valvulotomy for congenital aortic stenosis. Circulation 74 (Suppl. II), 2 (1986)
6. Lababidi Z, Weinhaus L: Successful balloon valvuloplasty for neonatal critical aortic stenosis. Am. Heart J. 112, 913 (1986)
7. Lababidi Z, Wu JR, Walls TJ: Percutaneous balloon aortic valvuloplasty: results in 23 patients. Am. J. Cardiol. 53, 194 (1984)
8. Neuhaus KL, Rupprath G: Ballondilatation kongenitaler Aortenstenosen. Z. Kardiol. 76 (Suppl. 6), 91 (1987)
9. Rupprath G, Neuhaus K-L: Percutaneous balloon valvuloplasty for aortic valve stenosis in infancy. Am. J. Cardiol. 55, 1655 (1985)
10. Rupprath G, Neuhaus K-L: Valvuloplastie der kongenitalen Aortenstenose. Herz 13, 14 (1988)
11. Sandor GGS, Olley PM, Trusler GA, Williams WG, Rowe RD, Morch JE: Long-term follow-up of patients after valvotomy for congenital valvular aortic stenosis in children. J. Thorac. Cardiovasc. Surg. 80, 171 (1980)
12. Sievert H, Kaltenbach M, Bussmann W-D, Kober G: Perkutane Valvuloplastik der Aortenklappe im Erwachsenenalter. DMW 111, 504 (1986)
13. Sievert H, Kober G, Bussmann W-D, Krämer P, Eckel L, Satter P, Kaltenbach M: Langzeitergebnisse der transluminalen Valvuloplastik bei verkalkter Aortenklappenstenose. DMW 113, 811 (1988)
14. Sievert H, Kober G, Reuhl I, Kaltenbach M, Bussmann W-D: Ergebnisse der Ballonvalvuloplastik bei valvulärer Pulmonalstenose. Herz 13, 20 (1988)
15. Vogel M, Benson LN, Freedom RM, Rowe RD: Balloon valvuloplasty for isolated aortic stenosis in children – short-term results. JACC 9, 130 A (1987)

Restenosis is a Common Feature of the Angiographic Follow-up After Balloon Valvoplasty of Calcified Aortic Stenoses

H. Sievert, P. Krämer, G. Kober, W.-D. Bussmann and M. Kaltenbach

Balloon dilatation of calcified aortic stenosis was attempted in 12 patients, 6 men and 6 women, aged 38–82 years. Two patients underwent emergency surgery because of myocardial injury or pericardial tamponade. One patient with severe depressed left ventricular function in whom the procedure was attempted in cardiogenic shock died during the procedure. One patient experienced severe aortic insufficiency after dilatation. The remaining pressure gradient was higher than 50 mmHg in another patient. Seven dilatations were considered to be successful with a remaining pressure gradient below 50 mmHg and a mean gradient reduction of 53 mmHg. In one of these 7 patients, who suffered from severe heart failure, valvoplasty had been carried out to make aortic valve replacement possible. The operation was performed 2 weeks later without complications. Five of 6 patients treated medically after successful valvoplasty had restenosis within 3 to 12 months. One of them exhibited a good result at 3 months but severe restenosis after one year. It is concluded that balloon valvoplasty of calcified aortic stenosis cannot be considered an alternative to surgery. If, however, left ventricular function improves after successful valvoplasty, valve replacement will then carry less risk.

Introduction

In January 1986, Cribier and his colleagues [1] reported three patients with calcified aortic stenosis in whom they performed balloon valvoplasty. Since that time, more than 1000 aortic valvoplasties have been reported worldwide [2–12]. In December 1984, we started percutaneous balloon valvoplasties for non-calcified adult aortic stenosis [13]. We extended the indications for this procedure in spring 1986 to include patients with severely calcified valves who were high risk candidates for surgery, or patients who preferred balloon dilatation [14, 15]. After successful procedures, the patients were monitored and recatheterized 3 to 6 months and 12 months later. In this presentation, we review those long-term results.

Patients

Balloon valvoplasty of calcified aortic stenosis was attempted in a total of 12 patients, 6 women and 5 men, between March 1986 and July 1987 and in one patient in March 1988. The mean age was 65 years, range 38–82 years. Nine of these patients were considered to be high risk surgical candidates due to age, severely depressed left ventricular function, breast cancer or pemphigus. One of these patients, a 57-year-old man, suffering from severe heart failure, had been operated three times because of mitral valvar disease and dysfunction of his mitral valvar prosthesis. Three patients were good candidates for surgery, but preferred balloon dilatation. One of these patients was referred to Rouen (France) after an unsuccessful attempt in Frankfurt and was reexamined in our department.

During the same time interval (between March 1986 and July 1987) 4 other high risk patients with calcified aortic stenosis were investigated in our hospital though not included in this study. In these patients, neither valvoplasty nor replacement of the aortic valve was performed for several reasons. All of them died within 6 months.

Methods

Valvoplasty procedure

All procedures were performed without premedication. A pigtail catheter was introduced into the aorta for pressure monitoring and an aortogram was performed to asess the severity of aortic insufficiency. Right heart catheterisation was performed in individual patients to determine the area of the aotric valve according to the Gorlin formula. A Sones catheter was then inserted into the ascending aortic through the other femoral artery (11 patients) or the brachial artery (one patient) and advanced via a straight guide wire into the left ventricle. The Sones catheter was exchanged for a balloon catheter. In the last 5 patients, a curved guide wire was employed to avoid myocardial injury which formed a large loop in the left ventricle. The diameter of the balloons ranged from 15–23 mm. In 3 patients, a 3×12 mm trefoil balloon catheter was used. The inflation time was, if possible, one minute. In patients in whom the arterial pressure showed a marked decrease, the balloon was inflated several times for a shorter period. For rapid deflation, the balloons were filled with diluted dye. After the last dilatation, the pressure recordings in the left ventricle and the aorta and the aortogram were repeated. 6 patients with a successful

Key words: Aortic stenosis; Valvoplasty; Balloon dilatation; Long-term results

Table 1. Acute clinical outcome

Patient no.	Sex	Age (years)	Aortic valve area (cm²)	Peak to peak gradient (mm Hg)	Complications
1	F	72	0.44 → 0.62	90 → 45	
2	M	64	0.85 → 1.44	100 → 40	
3*	M	38	0.68 → 1.58	90 → 10	
4	F	76	0.26 → 0.33	145 → 95	
5	F	65	0.44 → –	105 → 44	
6	M	41	0.64	120	myocardial injury
7	M	74	0.68	95	hemopericardium
8	F	74	0.34 → 0.56	60 → 15	
9	M	72	0.23	95	heart failure → died
10	F	82	0.46 → 0.7	60 → 20	
11	F	68	0.71 → 1.03	75 → 15	
12	M	57	0.48 → 0.87	60 → 35	

* Second attempt in Rouen/France

valvoplasty and a residual gradient after the procedure of less than 50 mmHg were reexamined by left heart catheterization (5 patients) or Doppler (1 patient) after 3 to 6 months and again after one year.

Results

Acute results

It was necessary in two patients to interrupt the procedure because of myocardial injury due to a straight exchange wire. One of them had a pericardial hematoma causing cardiac tamponade. The ofter had a myocardial hematoma without perforation of the ventricular wall. Valvar replacement was performed the same day in both cases. One of them, a 40-year-old man, recovered well, the other one, a 74-year-old high risk patient, experienced an apoplectic stroke two weeks later. In one patient with severely depressed left ventricular function, the procedure was done in cardiogenic shock. He died during the intervention although the dilatation was effective.

Balloon dilatation was possible in 9 patients without serious complications. All 9 experienced ventricular ectopic beats during inflation of the balloon. One patient transiently developed unconsciousness and one patient developed severe arterial hypotension without further consequences. In a 38-year-old patient, the brachial approach was used to introduce a 15 mm balloon catheter. The

pressure gradient remained nearly unchanged (90–80 mmHg). Some months later a second dilatation with a 23 mm balloon was performed in Rouen, France. The pressure gradient was reduced from 95 to 10 mmHg. This patient was reexamined two weeks later in our laboratory because of left ventricular failure. The pressure gradient had increased again to 75 mmHg and pulmonary artery pressure from normal to 55/20 mmHg. The aortogram showed severe regurgitation. At replacement of the valve, complete destruction of the left coronary leaflet was observed.

There was no increase in aortic regurgitation in the remaining 8 patients. Among these, there was one patient (no. 4) with a gradient of 145 mmHg before dilatation and a residual gradient of 95 mmHg after dilatation. This was not considered to be a success.

In the remaining 7 patients, the mean pressure gradient was reduced from 79 ± 20 to 26 ± 15 mmHg and was less than 50 mmHg in each case. These were considered successful dilatations. The area of the aortic valve had been determined in 6 of these patients, increasing from 0.6 ± 0,2 to 1,0 ± 0,4 cm². One of the 7 patients (no. 12), a 57-year-old man, who had been operated three times because of mitral valvar disease and dysfunction of the inserted mitral valve prostheses, and who suffered from a severe heart failure, had undergone valvoplasty to improve the clinical status. Replacement of the aortic valve was performed 2 weeks later without complications.

Long-term results

The dilatation was considered to be successful in 7 patients with a residual gradient after balloon dilatation of less than 50 mmHg (Fig. 1). 6 patients (nos. 1, 2, 5, 8, 10, 11) were re-examined after an interval of 3 to 12 months. In patient No 1, a 72-year-old woman, the gradient was reduced from 90 to 45 mmHg. Three months later the gradient had increased to 56 mmHg. Because of increasing severity of angina, successful surgery was performed with valvar replacement and aortocoronary bypass grafting. In a 64-year-old man (patient No. 2) the gradient had been reduced from 100 to 40 mmHg. Three months later,

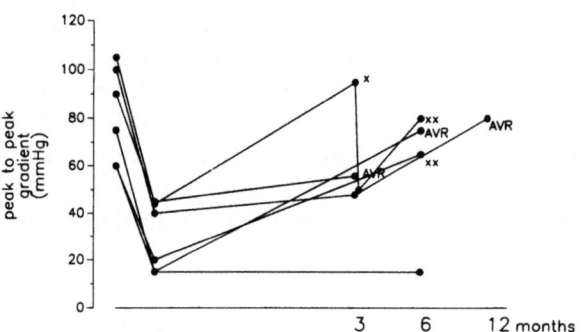

Fig. 1. Follow-up after successful valvoplasty. Five of 6 patients experienced sestenosis. × = second dilatation. × × = Doppler: AVR = aortic valve replacement

the gradient was 48 mmHg and one year later it had increased to 80 mmHg. In patient No. 5, a 65-year-old woman, suffering from advanced breast cancer, the gradient was reduced from 105 to 44 mmHg. Three months later the gradient had increased again to 95 mmHg. A second dilatation was performed, leaving a residual gradient of 50 mmHg. Three months later the gradient, measured by Doppler echocardiogram, had increased to 80 mmHg. In patient No. 8, a 74-year-old woman the gradient was reduced from 60 to 15 mmHg, but increased to 75 mmHg 6 months later. She refused surgery, because there was still some improvement in her clinical status. Patient No. 10, a 82-year-old woman whose gradient had been reduced from 60 to 20 mmHg refused recatheterization. Doppler echocardiography showed an increase of the pressure gradient to 65 mmHg after 6 months. In patient No. 11, a 68-year-old woman, in whom the pressure gradient was reduced from 75 to 15 mmHg, recatheterization at 4 months showed an unchanged favourable result with a residual gradient of 15 mmHg. Patient No. 12 was referred for surgery two weeks after successful valvoplasty.

Discussion

Since 1986, more than 1000 balloon dilatations of calcified aortic valves have been reported. With increasing experience and technical improvements, the complication rate has been reduced to 6% [2]. Balloon dilatation can lead to a dramatic improvement of the clinical status. Success rates up to 90% acutely have been reported [16, 17]. Recently, however, a high rate of restenosis has been demonstrated in non-invasive studies [10, 17–20]. Systematic angiographic follow-up studies, nonetheless, are unavailable. Only 23 of 500 patients (less than 5% of the French registry) have been re-examined by heart catheterization [21]. On the other hand, 8% of the patients were reported to have died within the first 4 months after the procedure [2, 3]. Most of these fatalities occurred in older patients who died at home. It is unknown, therefore, whether these patients had experienced restenosis.

The aortic pressure gradient was reduced below 50 mmHg (mean gradient reduction 53 mmHg) in only 8 of the 12 consecutive patients. One patient experienced severe aortic insufficiency. Only 7 dilatations, therefore, were considered to be successful. Six patients were followed and 5 of them experienced restenosis. Restenosis was found in 4 of them after intervals of 3 to 6 months and in one patient after one year. This patient had shown a good result at 3 months but severe restenosis developed by one year.

The mechanism of balloon dilatation of calcified aortic valves includes cracking of rigid calcifications within the valvar leaflets. The mobility of the valve leaflets can be restored partially in this fashion [8, 12, 22]. The process of restenosis may be explained either by a reaction to this destruction or by progression of the calcific process.

As a consequence of the described poor longterm results, balloon dilatation of calcified aortic valves cannot be considered a suitable alternative to valvar replacement. It may be indicated, however, in patients with cardiac failure and poor left ventricular function in whom surgery seems to be contra-indicated (as was the case in our patient No. 12). If left ventricular function improves after successful balloon dilatation, valvar replacement will then bear less risk.

References

1. Cribier A, Saoudi N, Berland J, Savin T, Rocha P, Letac B. Percutaneous transluminal valvuloplasty of acquired aortic stenosis in elderly patients: an alternative to valve replacement? Lancet 1986; 63–73

2. Berland J, Cribier A, Letac B, Guermonprey JL. Percutaneous aortic valvuloplasty in adults: immediate results of the French registry. Eur Heart J 1987; 8, (suppl 2): 241

3. Cribier A, Berland, J, Savin T. Mechmeche R, Saoudi N, Letac B. Percutaneous transluminal aortic valvuloplasty in adult aortic stenosis: results in 130 patients. J Am Coll Cardiol 1987; 9: 13A

4. Cribier A, Savin T, Berland J, et al. Percutaneous transluminal balloon valvuloplasty of adult aortic stenosis: report of 92 cases. J Am Coll Cardiol 1987; 9: 381–386

5. Erdmann E, Höfling B. Perkutane transfemorale Valvuloplastie der verkalkten und nicht verkalkten Aortenklappe. Dtsch Med Wochenschr 1987; 112: 1067–1072

6. Isner JM, Salem DN, Desnoyers MR, et al. Treatment of calcific aortic stenosis by balloon valvuloplasty. Am J Cardiol 1987; 59: 313–317

7. Jackson G, Thomas S, Monaghan M, Forsyth A, Jewit D. Inoperable aortic stenosis in the elderly: benefit from percutaneous transluminal valvuloplasty. Br Med J 1987; 294: 83–86

8. McKay RG, Safian RD, Lock JE et al. Balloon dilatation of calcified aortic stenosis in elderly patients: postmortem, intraoperative, and percutaneous valvuloplasty studies. Circulation 1986; 74: 119–125

9. Neuhaus KL. Aorten- und Mitralklappendilatationen. Vortrag Herbsttagung der Dtsch Ges f Herz- und Kreislaufforschung. Freiburg, 8–10 October 1987

10. Nishimura RA, Holmes DR, Reeder GS. Follow-up of patients undergoing percutaneous aortic balloon valvuloplasty by Doppler echocardiography. J Am Coll Cardiol 1988; 11: 234 A

11. Scherer HE, Hörmann E, Schwarten JU, Engel HJ. Perkutane Valvuloplastie verkalkter Aortenklappenstenosen: Alternative zum operativen Herzklappenersatz? Z Kardiol 1987; 76 (suppl 2): 59

12. Vahanian A, Guerinon J, Michel PL, Slama M, Grivaux M, Acar J. Experimental balloon valvuloplasty of calcified aortic stenosis in the elderly. Circulation 1986; 74 (suppl 11): 365

13. Sievert H, Kaltenbach M, Bussmann W-D., Kober G. Perkutane Valvuloplastik der Aortenklappe im Erwachsenenalter. Dtsch Med Wochschr. 1986; 111: 504–506

14. Bussmann W-D, Reifart N, Sievert H, Kaltenbach M. Transfemorale Valvuloplastik bei verkalkter Aortenklappenstenose. Dtsch Med Wochenschr 1987; 112: 723–725

15. Sievert H, Kober G, Kaltenbach M. Transluminale Valvuloplastik einer stenosierten und verkalkte Aortenklappe. Med Klinik 1986; 81: 855–857

16. Berman AD, Safian RD, Diver DJ, et al. Balloon aortic valvuloplasty of calcific aortic stenosis: results in 100 cases. Circulation 1987; 76 (suppl IV): 496

17. Bernard Y, Bassand JP, Anguenot T. et al. Early and late evaluation of percutaneous aortic valvuloplasty. A combined hemodynamic and doppler-echocardiographic study. J Am Coll Cardiol 1988; 11: 14 A

18. Berland J, Cribier A, Savin T. et al. Postvalvuloplasty follow-up of elderly patients with severe aortic stenosis and low ejection fraction. J Am Coll Cardiol 1988; 11: 15 A

19. Berman AD, Safian RD. Diver DJ, et al. Balloon aortic valvuloplasty of calcific aortic stenosis: results in 130 cases. J Am Coll Cardiol 1988; 11: 16 A

20. Lancelin B, Chevalier B, Bourdin T, et al. Mid-term follow-up after percutaneous transluminal aortic valvuloplasty in the elderly. J Am Coll Cardiol 1988; 11: 234 A

21. Letac B, Berland J, Mechmeche R, Savin T, Saoudi N, Cribier A. Late hemodynamic evaluation after percutaneous aortic valvuloplasty in adults with aortic stenosis. J Am Coll Cardiol 1987; 9: 14 A

22. Hamm CW, Langes K, Kupper W, Kalmar P, Bleifeld W. Morphologische Veränderungen bei Balloon-Valvuloplastie verkalkter Aortenklappenstenosen. Z Kardiol 1987; 76 (suppl 2): 21

Catheter Closure
of Patent Ductus

Ein Katheter zur Darstellung des Ductus arteriosus persistens

H. Sievert, E. Niemöller, W.-D. Bussmann, G. Kober, M. Kaltenbach,
mit technischer Assistenz von K. P. Köhler und W. Bamberg

A catheter for visualization of a patent ductus arteriosus

Summary: Nonsurgical technique for patent ductus closure require precise knowledge of ductus diameter, length and shape. Angiographic visualization, especially in adults, may be difficult, due to the high flow and overlap of the aorta or the pulmonary artery.
We have developed a new catheter for visualizing a patent ductus without intraarterial injection of contrast dye. A smooth latex balloon is mounted near the tip of this catheter and when it is filled with dye, the balloon fits the contours of the ductus.
Ductus diameter may be established by measuring the diameter of the balloon. Furthermore, the hemodynamic consequences of ductus closure may be observed with the balloon occluding the ductus.

Zusammenfassung: Für den nichtoperativen Verschluß des persistierenden Ductus Botalli ist es erforderlich, Durchmesser, Länge und Form des Duktus genau zu kennen. Da die angiographische Darstellung besonders bei Erwachsenen häufig unbefriedigend ist oder erst nach mehrfachen Kontrastmittelinjektionen eine überlagerungsfreie Darstellung gelingt, wurde ein Ballonkatheter zur Darstellung des offenen Duktus entwickelt.
Die Hülle des Ballons ist so weich und dehnbar, daß sie sich den Konturen des Duktus von innen anlegt, ohne einen nennenswerten Druck auf die Duktuswand auszuüben. Der Ballon wird im Duktus plaziert, mit Kontrastmittel gefüllt, gefilmt und vermessen.
Mit diesem Verfahren läßt sich der Duktus überlagerungsfrei darstellen. Kontrastmittel wird nur im Ballonkatheter appliziert. Die hämodynamischen Auswirkungen des Duktusverschlusses können vor dem Eingriff gemessen werden.

Einleitung

Die direkte angiographische Darstellung des Ductus arteriosus persistens ist wegen der hohen Strömungsgeschwindigkeit des Blutes und wegen Überlagerungen durch die Aorta und die Pulmonalarterie mitunter tech-

Schlüsselwörter: Duktus arteriosus persistens; Ductus Botalli
Key words: persistent ductus arteriosus

nisch schwierig (Abb. 1). Wir haben einen Latex-Ballonkatheter entwickelt, der eine sehr exakte indirekte Darstellung ohne Kontrastmittelbelastung ermöglicht. Zugleich können die hämodynamischen Auswirkungen eines Duktusverschlusses gemessen werden.

Methodik

Der zweilumige Duktusdarstellungs- und Okklusionskatheter (Edwards) trägt 3 cm proximal der Spitze einen 4 cm langen Ballon aus Latex. Der Durchmesser des Ballons beträgt in gefülltem Zustand 2 cm, entleert legt er sich dem 7F-Schaft so an, daß der Katheter durch eine 9F-Schleuse eingeführt werden kann. Die Ballonhülle ist sehr dehnbar, so daß der Druck im Ballon 0,5 bar nicht übersteigt. Eine durch den Ballon bewirkte Dilatation des Duktus ist deshalb ausgeschlossen.
Die Sondierung des Duktus erfolgt wie üblich über die Pulmonalarterie mit einem Cournand-Katheter oder über die Aora mit einem Duktus-Sondierungskatheter. Der Ballonkatheter wird über einen 0,035″-Wechseldraht in den Duktus eingeführt und mit Kontrastmittel gefüllt. Dabei legt sich die Ballonhülle der Duktuswand an, so daß die Form des Ballons der des Duktus entspricht. Durch Anwendung der Verschiebetechnik [2] oder – weniger genau – durch Vergleich mit dem Durchmesser des Katheterschaftes als Maßstab – können Durchmesser und Länge des Duktus gemessen werden. Während der Ballon den Duktus okkludiert, kann der Druck in der Arteria pulmonalis über das zentrale Lumen des Ballonkatheters gemessen werden, wenn der Katheter von der arteriellen Seite her eingeführt wird.

Ergebnisse

Mit konventioneller Technik unter Verwendung einer Hochdruckspritze (50 ml; 50 ml/s) ließ sich bei 10 von 40 Patienten im Alter von 11 bis 72 Jahren kein Angiogramm erzielen, das den Erfordernissen vor nicht chirurgischem Duktusverschluß voll entsprach.
Mit der neuen Technik ließ sich nach Sondierung des Duktus der Duktus-Darstellungskatheter problemlos über eine 9F-Schleuse einführen und im Duktus plazieren. Die Füllung erfolgte mit unverdünntem Kontrastmittel. Der Ballon ließ sich in gefülltem Zustand jeweils nur für kurze Zeit im Duktus halten. Er wurde deshalb in der Aorta gefüllt, dann langsam durch den Duktus in die Pulmonalarterie vorgeführt und dabei gefilmt (Abb.

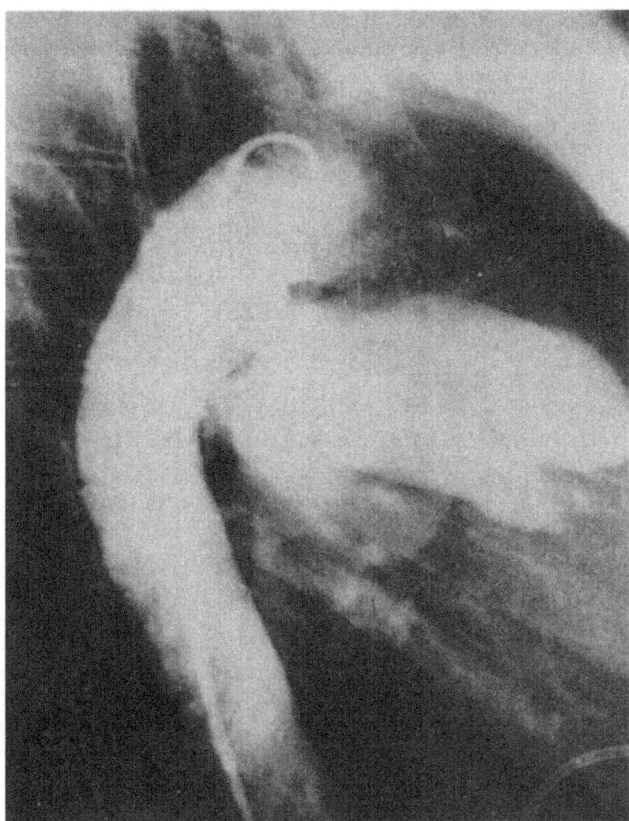

Abb. 1. Aortogramm im seitlichen Strahlengang: Großer Ductus Botalli mit massivem Kontrastmittelübertritt in die Pulmonalarterie. Der Duktus selbst ist jedoch schlecht abgrenzbar

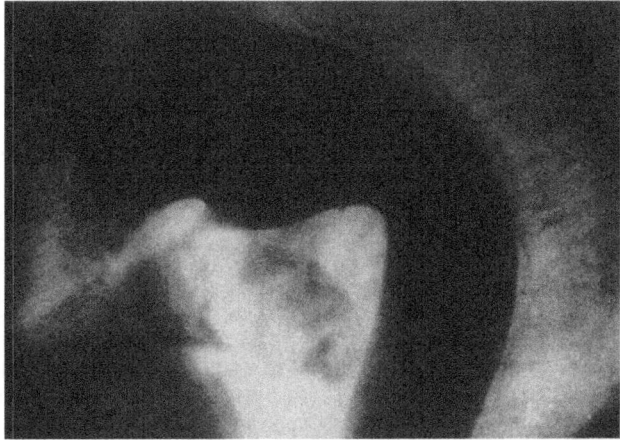

a

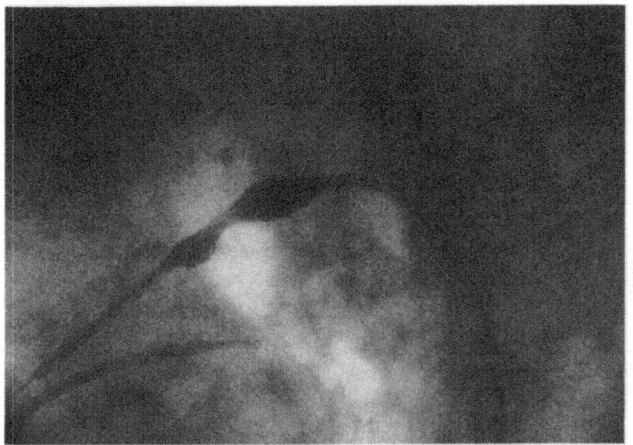

b

Abb. 2. Typischer Ductus Botalli, Darstellung angiographisch (**a**) und mit Spezialballonkatheter (**b**)

2a, b). Der Pulmonalarteriendruck konnte durch das zentrale Lumen gemessen werden.

Diskussion

Die Diagnose eines Ductus arteriosus persistens kann in den meisten Fällen durch die Auskultation gestellt werden. Seine hämodynamischen Auswirkungen lassen sich durch Indikatormethoden sowie Messungen der Drücke und der Sauerstoffsättigungswerte im großen und kleinen Kreislauf erfassen. Nuklearmedizinisch ist durch die Radionuklidventrikulographie eine nichtinvasive Quantifizierung möglich [3]. Als Voraussetzung für nichtoperative Verschlußtechniken [1, 4–6] ist eine exakte Bestimmung von Durchmesser, Länge und Form des Duktus erforderlich. Bei Patienten mit pulmonaler Hypertonie sollte darüber hinaus eine Messung der hämodynamischen Auswirkungen des Duktusverschlusses vor Durchführung des verschließenden Eingriffes erfolgen.

In vielen Fällen kann der Duktus durch eine Aortographie im seitlichen Strahlengang dargestellt werden. Hierzu muß eine große Kontrastmittelmenge (50 ml) in sehr kurzer Zeit (1 s) injiziert werden. Die Aufnahmefrequenz muß wenigstens 6 Bilder/s betragen. Bei sehr hoher Strömungsgeschwindigkeit im Duktus kann jedoch die angiographische Darstellung so schwierig sein, daß nach Lagekorrektur des Katheters mehrfache Kontrastmittelinjektionen durchgeführt werden müssen. Schließlich gibt

es Fälle, in denen der Duktus z. B. durch eine stark elongierte Aorta und die erweiterte Pulmonalarterie so überlagert ist, daß er nicht frei projiziert werden kann. Dies kommt besonders bei älteren Patienten vor (Abb. 1). Auch in diesen Fällen kann mit dem beschriebenen Spezialkatheter der Duktus überlagerungsfrei und ohne Kontrastmittelinjektion sehr genau dargestellt werden.

Bei Patienten mit pulmonaler Hypertonie und besonders bei Druckangleich zwischen großem und kleinem Kreislauf ist es von großer praktischer Bedeutung, die Auswirkungen eines Duktusverschlusses auf den Kreislauf zu kennen. Allgemein gilt ein Duktusverschluß nur dann als indiziert, wenn der Druck in der Arteria pulmonalis nach dem Verschluß abfällt. Die funktionelle Auswirkung eines Duktusverschlusses läßt sich mit dem hier beschriebenen Verfahren vorab bestimmen. Wenn die Ballonokklusion bei gekreuztem Shunt zu einer weiteren Steigerung des Pulmonalisdruckes führt, ist der Duktusverschluß kontraindiziert.

Eine weitere technische Verbesserung des Katheters ist vorgesehen. Sie besteht in einer Versteifung des Katheterschaftes und einer Vorbiegung, die es ermöglicht, daß der Duktus direkt sondiert werden kann.

Nachtrag bei der Korrektur: Inzwischen ist eine verbesserte Version des Katheters mit einer Vorbiegung und einem weiteren Lumen zur Messung des Aortendruckes erhältlich (Fa. Edwards).

Literatur

1. Bussmann W-D, Sievert H, Kaltenbach M (1984) Transfemoraler Verschluß des Ductus arteriosus persistens. Dtsch med Wochenschr 109: 1322
2. Kaltenbach M, Schul W (1975) Kineangriographische Bestimmung von Ventrikelvolumina mit Rechnerhilfe. Dtsch med Wochenschr 10: 590
3. Klepzig H, Sievert H, Standke R, Mildenberger D, Bussmann W-D, Hör G, Kaltenbach M (1987) Nuklearmedizinische Shunt-Bestimmung beim Ductus arteriosus Botalli. Nuklearmedizin 26: 33
4. Porstmann W, Wierny L, Warnke H (1967) Der Verschluß des Ductus arteriosus persistens ohne Thorakotomie. Thoraxchirurgie 15: 199
5. Rashkind WJ (1983) Transcatheter treatment of congenital heart disease. Circulation 67: 711
6. Sievert H, Bussmann W-D, Kaltenbach M (1987) Closure of leftto-right shunts by catheter techniques. In: Hilger HH, Hombach V, Rashkind WJ (eds) Invasive Cardiovascular Therapy. Martinus Nijhoff Publishers, Dordrecht Boston Lancaster, pp 25–38

Eingegangen 29. Dezember 1987
akzeptiert 10. Februar 1988

Für die Verfasser:
Dr. H. Sievert, Abteilung für Kardiologie, Zentrum der Inneren Medizin, Universitätsklinikum, Theodor-Stern-Kai 7, 6000 Frankfurt 70

Visualization of the Patent Ductus by Means of a new low Pressure Balloon Catheter

H. Sievert, E. Niemöller, W.-D. Bussmann, G. Kober and M. Kaltenbach

A new angiographic method of determining the anatomy of a patent ductus arteriosus (PDA) preparatory to its surgical or nonsurgical closure has been developed and compared to conventional angiographic techniques in 17 patients using a new low pressure balloon catheter (Edwards). The balloon, 5 cm long, is filled with contrast material and expanded to any diameter up to 20 mm. It may be passed into the ductus from either the arterial (14 patients) or venous (3 patients) side. The balloon is expanded by radiopaque material adjacent to the aortic orifice of the PDA and advanced (or pulled) through the ductus. Deformation of the balloon identified the lenght and caliber of the PDA providing virtually identical estimates there of in all 17 patients when compared to conventional angiography. On the other hand, visualization of the PDA was good in only 41 (62%) or tolerable in 14 (21%) of 66 conventionally studied patients. (J Interven Cardiol 1988: 1:2)

Introduction

Accurate visualization of the patent ductus is desirable before surgical closure. Before nonsurgical closure the length and diameter of the ductus must be determined to provide adequate occluding devices [1–6]. If the ductus is to be occluded with an ivalon plug, it is mandatory to determine the shape, length and the diameter of the plug before the procedure to guarantee complete occlusion of the ductus and reliable plug fixation [1, 3, 6]. In patients with severe pulmonary hypertension it is also important to measure pulmonary artery (PA) pressure during provisional ductus occlusion.

With conventional angiography adequate ductus opacification can be difficult since the contrast material is quickly washed out and satisfactory density may not be achieved despite the injection of 50 mL contrast material with a flow rate of 40 to 60 mL/s. A further disadvantage is that some patients present with an overlapping aorta and/or pulmonary artery. A new method for visualizing the patent ductus has therefore been developed.

Patients

From June 1983 to May 1988 catheterization of patent ductus arteriosus (PDA) was carried out in 66 patients. Nineteen were males and 47 females, the mean age was 41 ± 18 years (range 8 to 73 years). In 10 patients fluoroscopy showed calcification of the ductus. In all patients the purpose of the study was to perform exact measurements of the ductus diameter as a prerequisite for transfemoral ductus closure.

Methods

Angiography. Right heart catheterization was performed using conventional techniques. A high flow pigtail catheter was introduced percutaneously into the common femoral artery, according to the Seldinger technique, after which the patient received 100 U/kg of heparin. The catheter was advanced to the descending part of the aortic arch and 50 mL of contrast material were injected with a flow rate of 50 mL/s. The images were taken in the lateral projection at a cine speed of 50 frames/s. If the PDA was not clearly visible, additional injections were recorded in LAO- and RAO-projections. If necessary, caudal and/or cranial projections were chosen. For calibration a previously described technique [7] was used. The catheter was filmed before and after moving the x-ray table a distance of 6 cm. The quality of ductus visualization was graded as good, tolerable or insufficient.

Low Pressure Balloon Catheter. In addition to conventional angiography a new low pressure balloon catheter (Edwards) was employed in the last 17 patients. It is a 7.5 French end hole catheter with a second lumen leading into a latex-balloon. The balloon, 5 cm long, is mounted 7 cm proximal of the tip of the catheter. It is filled with contrast material (Urografine^R) and can be expanded by low pressure (0.5 atm above environmental pressure) to any diameter up to 20 mm. The central lumen of the catheter accepts an 0.035" exchange wire and may be used for pressure measurement. The tip of the catheter is preshaped as shown in Figure 1. A revised version of the catheter provides a third lumen for pressure measurements proximal of the balloon, i.e. in the aorta, when the catheter is introduced from the arterial side.

The catheter was inserted through a 9 French sheet. In 3 patients, it was introduced using an exchange wire after entering the PDA with a preshaped multipurpose catheter. In 11 patients it was advanced to the descending aorta using an 0.035" J-wire. After removal of the wire, the patent ductus was entered with the balloon catheter. In another three patients, the catheter was introduced over an exchange wire from the venous side. In these patients, the patent ductus was approached via the pulmonary artery with a multipurpose catheter and a straight guide wire. After insertion of the low pressure balloon catheter

Reprint from J of Interventional Cardiology, 1 (No. 2), 143–148, 1986, Futura Pub. Mount Kisco

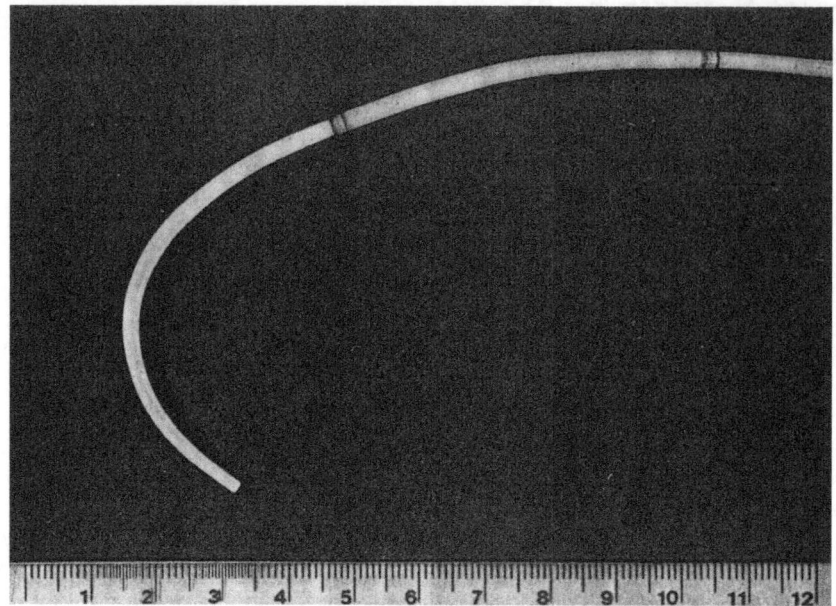

Fig. 1. Due to the preshaped tip of the catheter the patent ductus can easily be entered via the descending aorta

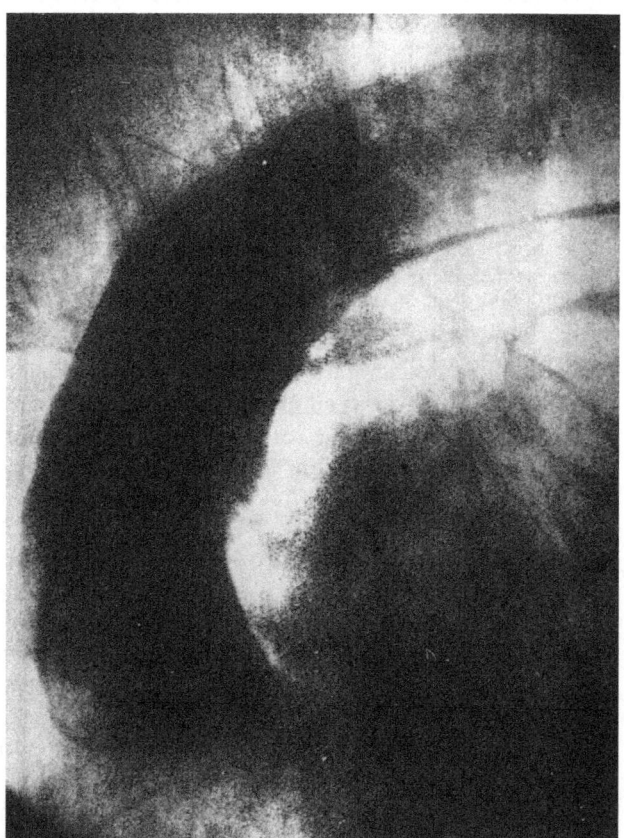

Fig. 2. a Lateral aortogram of a 72-year-old woman showed opacification of the pulmonary artery. The patent ductus is not clearly visibly

into the PDA, the balloon was positioned in the descending aorta and filled with contrast material. The balloon was slowly advanced (or pulled, when introduced from the venous side) to the aortic orifice of the ductus. The contrast material in the balloon was slowly removed, until the balloon slipped into the pulmonary artery with minimal resistance. Simultaneous filming (cine speed: 50 frames/s) showed the contours of the balloon clearly outlining the ductus including its widened entrance at the aortic side.

In patients with pulmonary hypertension, pulmonary artery pressure during ductus occlusion was measured by way of keeping the balloon in the PDA or the widened entrance on the aortic side.

Results

Angiography. Angiography was performed in 66 patients. Additional injections of contrast material in other projections were necessary in 30 patients. The visualization of the PDA was good in 41 patients, tolerable in 14 patients and insufficient in 11 patients.

Low Pressure Balloon Catheter. The balloon catheter was used in the last 17 consecutive patients. In 14 of them it was introduced via the femoral artery, in three patients via the femoral vein.

Inserting the catheter into the ductus was possible without any problems or complications in all patients. In all of them the PDA was clearly visualized by the balloon (Figs. 2A and B). Pulmonary artery pressure measurements (Fig. 3) were performed in three patients with pulmonary hypertension, demonstrating a pressure decrease in two of them during provisional ductus occlusion.

In 13 of the 17 patients, in whom the balloon catheter was used, the conventional angiogram was considered to be of good or tolerable quality. With conventional angiography, the mean ductus diameter in these 13 patients was 5.0 ± 3 mm, and 4.9 ± 2.9 using the balloon technique. In 4 patients the opacification was considered insufficient due to overlapping structures.

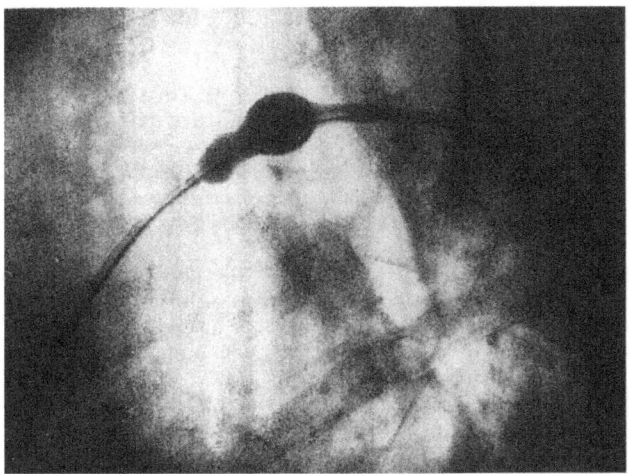

Fig. 2. b The ductus diameter could easily be measured using the new low pressure balloon catheter

Discussion

Our experience with patent ductus in 66 patients (19 male, 47 female, aged 8 to 73 years) has shown that opacification obtained with conventional angiographic techniques was not adequate in the case of 11 patients to determine the diameter, length and shape of the ductus before nonsurgical closure. Eight of the 66 patients had pulmonary hypertension making PA pressure measurements during provisional occlusion desirable. The new method was proven to be accurate and easy to handle in the case of 17 patients. It appears superior to conventional angiography, particularly in patients with difficult opacification or overlap of other structures with the ductus. An additional advantage of this technique is that direct injection of contrast material with concurrent side effects is avoided. Further improvement in catheter design should allow introduction through an 8 F or 7 F sheath.

There is good evidence for no risk in using this balloon technique. The filling pressure of the balloon is too low to cause any damage to the PDA. However, the catheter should not be introduced into a PDA with a diameter smaller than the catheter. Furthermore, the balloon should not be pulled back to the pulmonary artery with force. Maneuvering the balloon without resistance or with minimal resistance is always possible, if the contrast material in the balloon is slowly withdrawn. Until now, we have no experience in using this technique in the case of patent ductus with aneurysm. One can expect, however, that large aneurysms of patent ductus cannot be visualized by this technique.

Beyond opacification of the patent ductus, the described technique may be used for the opacification of other high flow structures, such as ventricular septal defects, aortico-pulmonary defects, atrial septal defects or arterio-venous fistulas, though we have no experience with this technique in these particular lesions. The catheter and especially the balloon has of course to be adequately modified when applied to the opacification of other cardiovascular defects. The use of this balloon technique may become increasingly important with the refinement of catheter techniques for nonoperative closure procedures [8, 9].

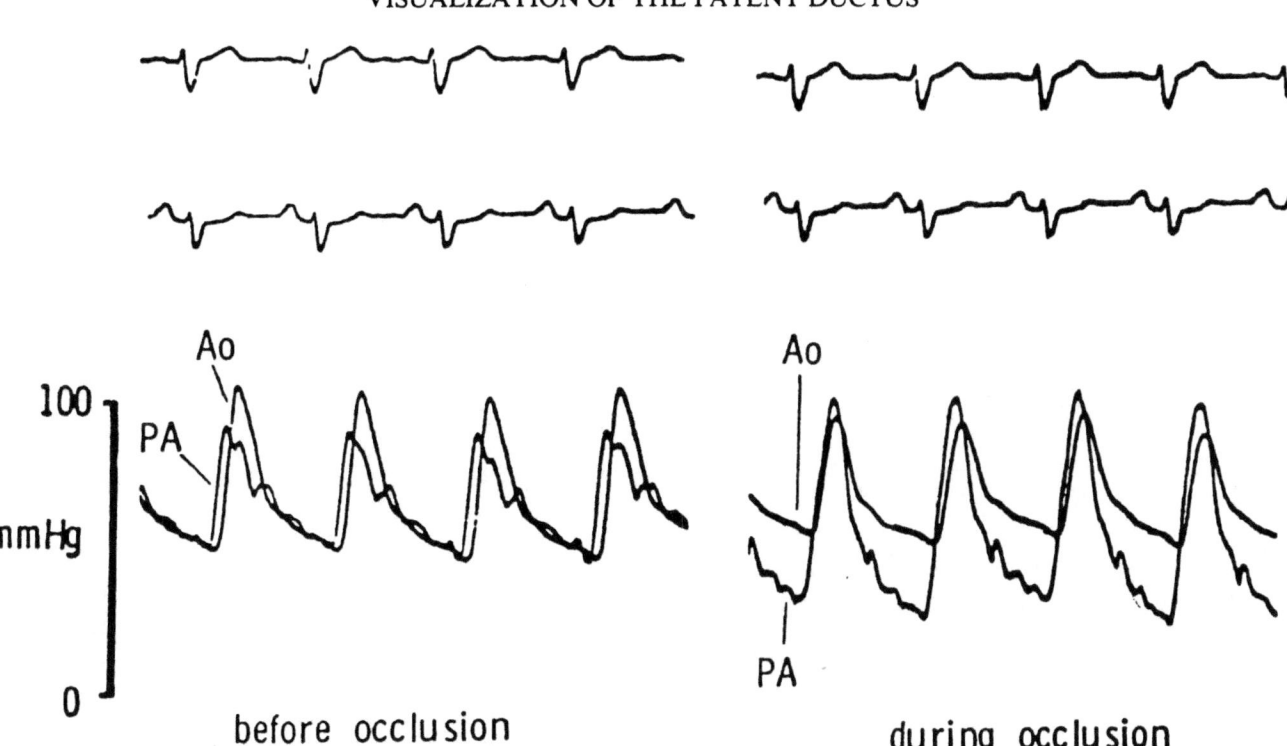

VISUALIZATION OF THE PATENT DUCTUS

Fig. 3. In a 61-year-old man with severe pulmonary hypertension, due to a large persistent ductus arteriosus, provisional ductus occlusion led to a marked decrease in diastolic pulmonary artery pressure, while systolic pulmonary artery pressure increased

Reprint from J of Interventional Cardiology, 1 (No. 2), 143–148, 1986,
Futura Pub. Mount Kisco

Summary

Nonsurgical techniques for patent ductus closure require precise knowledge of ductus diameter, length and shape. Angiographic visualization may be difficult due to high flow and overlap of the aorta or pulmonary artery.

We have developed a new low pressure balloon catheter for visualizing a patent ductus without need for contrast injection. Near the tip of this catheter a smooth latex balloon is mounted, which, filled with contrast material, fits the contours of the ductus. Ductus diameter may be assessed by measuring the diameter of the balloon and the hemodynamic consequences of ductus closure may be observed by measuring pulmonary artery pressure with the balloon occluding the ductus. This balloon catheter was used in 17 patients without any complications. Visualization of the ductus was excellent in all of them. Pulmonary artery pressure measurements in three patients with pulmonary hypertension showed a pressure decrease during provisional ductus occlusion in two of them.

After technical refinement, the low pressure balloon catheter may be employed in visualizing other high flow structures such as ventricular septal defects or aortico-pulmonary septal defects.

References

1. Bussmann W-D, Sievert H, Kaltenbach M. Transfemoraler Verschluß des Ductus arteriosus persistens. Dtsch med Wschr 1984; 109: 1322
2. Endrys J, Simo M, Valliattu J, Yousof A, Khan N, Zanaouma Y. New technique of percutaneous closure of patent ductus arteriosus by a detachable balloon. Circulation 1987; 76 (Suppl IV): 45 ·
3. Porstmann W, Wierny L, Warnke H. Der Verschluß des Ductus arteriosus persistens ohne thorakotomie. Thoraxchirurgie 1967; 15: 199
4. Rashkind WJ. Transcatheter treatment of congenital heart disease. Circulation 1983; 67: 711–716
5. Sievert H, Bussmann WD, Kaltenbach M. Closure of left-to-right shunts by catheter techniques. In Hilger HH, Hombach V, Rashkind WJ (eds): Invasive Cardiovascular Therapy. Dordrecht-Boston-Lancaster Martinus Nijhoff Publishers, 1987, pp. 25–38
6. Sievert H, Niemöller E, Köhler KP, Bamberg W, Hanke H, Satter P, Kaltenbach M, Bussmann W-D. Langzeitergebnisse des transfemoralen Ductus-Botalli-Verschlusses. Dtsch med Wschr 1988; (in press)
7. Kaltenbach M, Schulz W. Kineangiographische Bestimmung von Ventrikelvolumina mit Rechnerhilfe. Dtsch med Wschr 1975; 100: 590
8. Latson LA, Sobczyk WL, Kilzer KJ, McManns BM. Closure of atrial septal defects with the Rashkind occluder. Circulation 1987; 76 (Suppl IV): 265
9. Lock JE, Block PC, McKay RG, Baim DS, Keane JF. Catheter closure of postinfarction/postoperative ventricular defects: initial experience. Circulation 1987; 76 (Suppl IV): 28

Transfemoraler Ductus-Botalli-Verschluß

Akut- und Langzeitergebnisse

H. Sievert, E. Niemöller, K. P. Köhler, W. Bamberg, H. Hanke, P. Satter, M. Kaltenbach und W.-D. Bussmann

Bei 38 Patienten im mittleren Alter von 39 (11–72) Jahre wurde ein Ductus arterious persistens mit einem transfemoral eingeführten Ivalon-Pfropfen verschlossen. Der Durchmesser des Ductus betrug im Mittel 4,5 ± 1,2 (2–9) mm, der Druck in der Pulmonalarterie im Mittel 30/12 (15/5–70/27) mmHg. Bei zwei Patienten kam es ohne schwerwiegende Folgen nach 2 bzw. 7 Wochen zu einer Pfropfdislokation. In allen anderen Fällen konnte der Ductus erfolgreich verschlossen werden. Die Komplikationsrate war niedrig, schwere Komplikationen traten nicht auf. Im Langzeitverlauf kam es bei einer Nachbeobachtungszeit bis zu 4 Jahren zu keiner Rekanalisation des Ductus oder Dislokation des Pfropfes.

Transfemoral catheter closure of persistent ductus arteriosus

A persistent ductus arteriosus was occluded with an Ivalon plug via a catheter delivery system, introduced through the femoral artery, in 38 patients, aged 11–72 years (mean 39). The mean diameter of the ductus was 4.5 ± 1.2 (2–9) mm, mean pulmonary artery pressure 30/12 (15/5–70/27) mmHg. In two patients the plug became dislocated after two and seven weeks, respectively, without serious consequences. In all others the occlusion was successful and permanent. There were only a few complications and none was serious. During a follow-up period of up four years there were no instances of recanalization or further plug dislocation.

Der Ductus arteriosus persistens ist die häufigste angeborene Mißbildung des Herz-Kreislauf-Systems. Infolge des Links-Rechts-Shunts von der Aorta zur Pulmonalarterie kommt es zu einer Hyperzirkulation im kleinen Kreislauf. Mögliche Spätfolgen sind eine Linksherzinsuffizienz oder eine Rechtsherzinsuffizienz infolge einer reaktiven pulmonalen Hypertonie – unter Umständen bis hin zum Druckangleich zwischen großem und kleinem Kreislauf (Eisenmenger-Reaktion). Gefürchtet ist ferner eine bakterielle Endokarditis bzw. Aortitis, deren Häufigkeit in der Literatur mit 2–8% angegeben wird [3, 13]. Wegen dieser möglichen Spätfolgen wird in jedem Fall ein Ductus-Verschluß angestrebt. Im Neugeborenenalter wird dies durch die Gabe von Prostaglandinsynthesehemmern versucht [4, 5, 17], welche zu einer Kontraktion der glatten Muskulatur in der Ductus-Wand führen können. Jenseits des Neugeborenenalters wird üblicherweise ein operativer Verschluß durchgeführt.

Bereits 1967 beschrieben Porstmann und Mitarbeiter [20] eine Technik des nicht-operativen Ductus-Verschlusses mit einem über die Femoralarterie eingeführten Propf aus Ivalon. Dieses Verfahren konnte sich jedoch bisher nicht allgemein durchsetzen und wurde nur von Kliniken in Japan [11, 26, 29] und China [23] übernommen. Wir haben erstmals 1983 mit dieser Methode einen Ductus Botalli verschlossen [2, 27]. Im folgenden berichten wir über die Akut- und Langzeitergebnisse bei 38 Patienten.

Patienten und Methodik

Patienten. Ein transfemoraler Ductus-Botalli-Verschluß wurde bei 38 Patienten, 27 Frauen und 11 Männern im Alter von 11 bis 72 Jahren (Durchschnittsalter 39 Jahre), vorgenommen. Bei 17 Patienten wurde die Diagnose im Rahmen einer Routineuntersuchung gestellt. Bei den anderen gaben Atemnot bei körperlicher Belastung (n = 13), Knöchelödeme (n = 2), eine allgemeine Leistungsminderung (n = 6), Herzrhythmusstörungen (n = 5) oder andere uncharakteristische Beschwerden (n = 8) Anlaß zu einer ärztlichen Untersuchung. Bei fünf Patienten wurde zu einem früheren Zeitpunkt eine Endokarditis bzw. Septikämie diagnostiziert. Bei drei Patienten war ein operativer Verschluß ohne bleibenden Erfolg vorausgegangen.

In den meisten Fällen war ein typisches systolisch-diastolisches Maschinengeräusch auskultierbar, bei einzelnen Patienten war das Geräusch sehr diskret. Elektrokardiographisch wiesen 34 Patienten einen Sinusrhythmus, die übrigen vier Patienten Vorhofflimmern auf. Das röntgenologisch bestimmte Herzvolumen war bei 20 von 29 Patienten vergrößert (obere Normgrenze 700 ml/1,73 m² bei Frauen 800 ml/173 m² bei Männern) und betrug im Mittel 937 ± 332 ml/1,73 m² (n = 29). Der Pulmonalarteriendruck war bei zehn Patienten normal, bei elf grenzwertig und bei 17 Patienten erhöht; er betrug im Mittel 30 ± 8 zu 12 ± 5 mmHg. Der anhand einer peripheren Farbstoffverdünnungskurve berechnete Links-Rechts-Shunt betrug zwischen unter 20 und mehr als 60% des Herzzeitvolumens im kleinen Kreislauf, im Mittel 30%. In keinem Fall lag ein wesentlicher Rechts-Links-Shunt vor. Der angiographisch bestimmte Durchmesser des Ductus betrug zwischen 2 und 9 mm, im Mittel 4,5 ± 1,2 mm.

Methodik. Zunächst wurde der Ductus angiographisch dargestellt. Hierzu wurde ein Aortogramm im seitlichen Strahlengang angefertigt. Um eine ausreichende Kontrastmittelanfärbung des Ductus zu erzielen, war eine Injektion von 50 ml Kontrastmittel mit einem Fluß von 50

ml/s erforderlich. Aus dem Angiogramm wurde mit Hilfe der Verschiebetechnik [10] der Durchmesser des Ductus gemessen. Anschließend erfolgte eine Beckenübersichts-angiographie zur Bestimmung des Durchmessers der Bek-ken- bzw. Femoralarterien. In der letzten Zeit erfolgte die Ductus-Darstellung mit einer neuen Technik [28]: Da-bei wird ein Katheter mit einem kontrastmittelgefüllten,

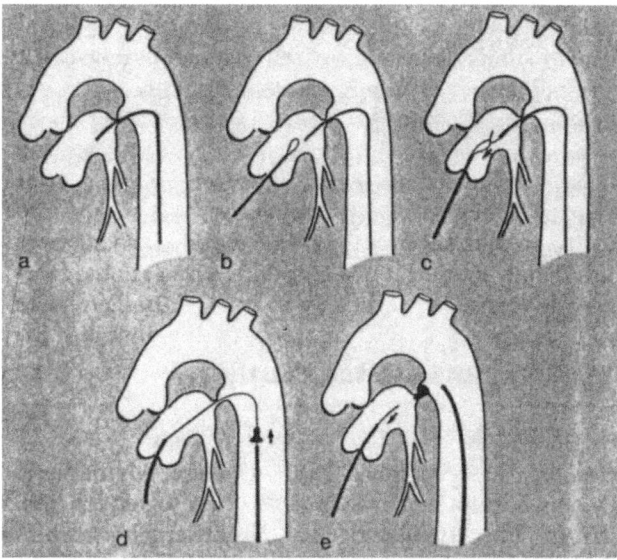

Abb. 1. Der Ductus wird von der Aorta aus mit einem vorgebogenen Katheter sondiert (**a**). Über die Vena femoralis wird ein 10F-Kathe-ter in die Pulmonalarterie gelegt. Durch diesen Katheter wird eine Drahtschlinge eingeführt (**b**). Mit ihr wird ein durch den arteriellen Katheter eingeführter 4 m langer Draht gefangen und zur venösen Seite herausgezogen (**c**). Nach Austausch des arteriellen Katheters gegen einen großlumigen Applikator wird ein Ivalon-Pfropf auf den Applikator aufgefädelt und in den Ductus vorgeschoben (**d**). Nach Verankerung des Pfropfes im Ductus wird die Drahtschiene entfernt (**e**)

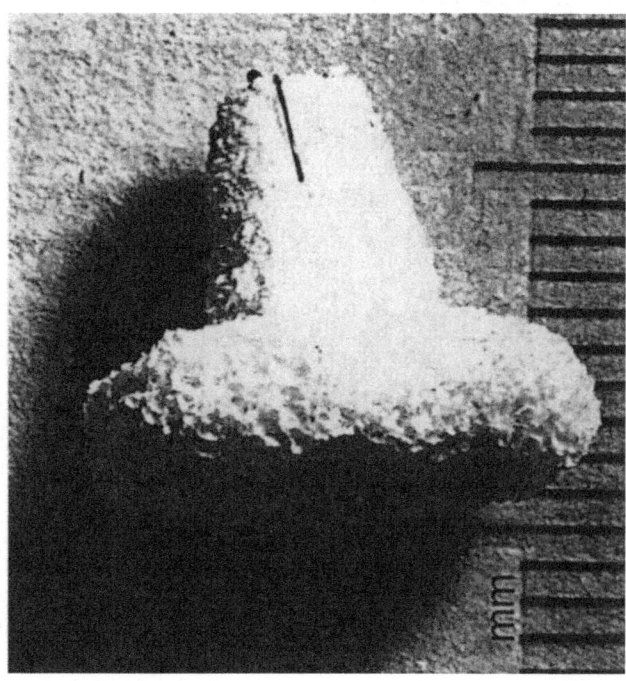

Abb. 2. Ivalon-Pfropf

sehr weichen Latex-Ballon in den Ductus geführt. Der Ballon paßt sich den Konturen des Ductus an, wird ge-filmt und vermessen.

Der eigentliche Ductus-Verschluß erfolgte in einer zwei-ten Sitzung (Abbildung 1). Entsprechend der Form und Größe des Ductus wurde aus Ivalon® ein Pfropf angefer-tigt (Abbildung 2). Zur Stabilisierung wurde er auf ein Stahlgerüst aus 0,5 mm starkem Edelstahl aufgezogen. Die Fixierung an diesem Stahlgerüst erfolgte durch Hal-tefäden an der Spitze des Pfropfes. Zur Auffädelung auf eine Drahtschiene wurde der Pfropf mit einer zentralen Bohrung versehen.

Nach Lokalanästhesie wurde eine Femoralvene punktiert und ein 10F-Katheter in die Pulmonalarterie geführt. Die Sondierung des Ductus erfolgte von der arteriellen Seite mit einem stark vorgebogenen 7F-Katheter. Durch ihn wurde eine 4 m langer Drahtschiene mit flexibler Spitze in die Pulmonalaterie geführt und dort mit einer über den venösen Katheter eingeführten Schlinge gefangen. Mit der Schlinge wurde die Drahtschiene zur venösen Seite durchgezogen. Auf diese arterio-transduktal-venöse Drahtschiene konnte der Ivalon-Pfropf aufgefädelt wer-den. Zuvor mußte die arterielle Punktionsstelle mit einem Dilatator erweitert und eine Einführschleuse (Applika-tor) in die Femoralarterie gelegt werden. Der Durchmes-ser dieses Applikators betrug je nach Größe des Pfropfes zwischen 5,2 und 9 mm. Der Ivalon-Pfropf wurde mit einer ebenfalls auf den Draht aufgefädelten 20 cm langen, an der Spitze stumpfen Kanüle durch den Applikator bis in die Beckenarterie vorgeschoben. Anschließend wurde der Pfropf mit einem speziellen Schiebekatheter bis in den Ductus gebracht. Die korrekte Plazierung des Pfrop-fes war durch eine Einkerbung zu erkennen und wurde durch eine Kontrastmittelinjektion nachgewiesen. An-schließend wurde die 4 m lange Drahtschiene über die venöse Seite herausgezogen.

Bei acht Patienten wurde wegen einer im Verhältnis zum Applikator relativ zu kleinen Fermoralarterie das Gefäß vor der Punktion operativ freigelegt. In diesen Fällen wurde nach dem Eingriff die Arterie durch eine fortlau-fende Naht verschlossen. In allen übrigen Fällen erfolgte die Blutstillung durch manuelle Kompression und einem Druckverband für 24 Stunden.

Ergebnisse

In allen Fällen konnte eine arterio-transduktal-venöse Drahtschiene gelegt und ein Ivalon-Pfropf eingeführt werden. Bei drei Patienten war der Pfropf im Verhältnis zum Ductus zu klein und ließ sich ohne großen Wider-stand in die Pulmonalarterie schieben. Er wurde weiter bis in die Femoralvene vorgeschoben und dort operativ in Lokalanästhesie entfernt. In gleicher Sitzung wurde über die noch liegende Drahtschiene der Ductus mit ei-nem größeren Pfropfen verschlossen. In allen anderen Fällen ließ sich der zuerst eingeführte Pfropf im Ductus plazieren. Die Blutstillung an der Punktionsstelle erfolgte durch manuelle Kompression. Bei einem Patienten wurde einige Stunden nach dem Eingriff eine Nachblutung durch operative Naht des Gefäßes versorgt. Bei einer Patientin mit einem Ductus-Durchmesser von 8 mm und einer 8 mm dicken Femoralarterie wurde am Tag nach dem Eingriff wegen eines thrombotischen Verschlusses der Arterie eine operative Thrombektomie erforderlich.

Der Ductus-Verschluß wurde angiographisch sowie durch Auskultation, Farbstoffverdünnungskurven und das Röntgenbild mit der typischen Position des Pfropfes nachgewiesen (Abbildung 3).

Bei acht Patienten entwickelten sich einige Tage nach dem Ductus-Verschluß subfebrile Temperaturen (~ 38 °C), ohne daß in den daraufhin zahlreich entnommenen Blutkulturen ein Erreger nachgewiesen werden konnte. In allen Fällen normalisierte sich die Körpertemperatur einige Tage später spontan. Diejenigen Patienten, die vor dem Ductus-Verschluß unter mehr oder weniger ausgeprägter Atemnot litten, gaben eine deutliche Besserung an. In diesen Fällen fand sich bereits wenige Tage nach dem Ductus-Verschluß eine eindrucksvolle Rückbildung der Lungenstauung und Abnahme der Herzgröße (Abbildung 4). Die Patienten wurden wenige Tage nach dem Eingriff aus der stationären Behandlung entlassen und in regelmäßigen Abständen (nach 3 Monaten, 1 Jahr, 3–4 Jahren) zu Nachuntersuchungen einbestellt.

Bei zwei Patienten kam es 2 bzw. 7 Wochen nach dem Ductus-Verschluß zu einer Dislokation des Pfropfes in die

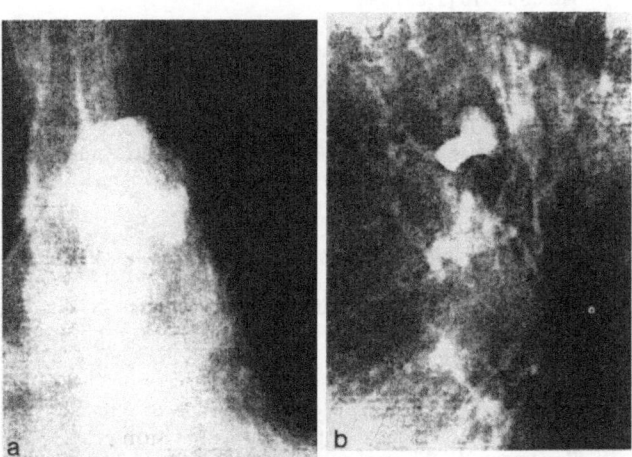

Abb. 3. Eine Ausschnittvergrößerung zeigt den Ivalon-Pfropf in typischer Position. **a** Strahlengang posterior-anterior, **b** seitlicher Strahlengang

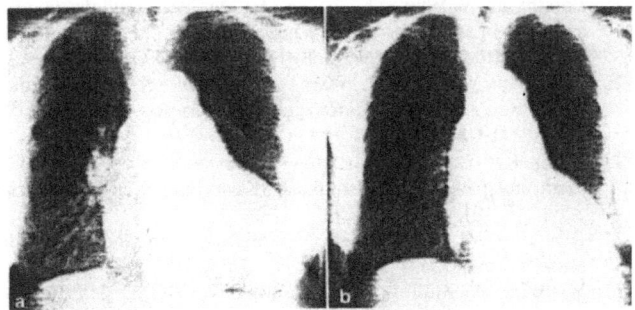

Abb. 4. Röntgenaufnahme des Thorax vor (**a**) und einen Tag nach (**b**) transfemoralem Ductus-Verschluß mit einem Ivalon-Pfropf: Rückbildung von Lungenstauung und Herzgröße

Pulmonalarterie, ohne daß dies zu einer gravierenden klinischen Symptomatik geführt hätte. Im einen Fall – es handelte sich um einen 51jährigen, 6 Jahre zuvor erfolglos operierten Patienten – wurde der Ductus operativ durch eine Patch-Plastik verschlossen und der Pfropf aus der Pulmonalarterie entfernt. Bei dem anderen Patienten erfolgte der Ductus-Verschluß einige Monate später durch einen zweiten Ivalon-Pfropf. Der zuerst eingeführte Pfropf okkludierte einen Ast der Pulmonalarterie und wurde dort belassen. Nach diesen Erfahrungen wurden die Pfröpfe 20–30 % größer als dem Ductus-Durchmesser entsprechend gewählt. Danach kam es zu keinen weiteren Pfropfdiskolationen.

14 Patienten wurden länger als ein Jahr, sieben Patienten länger als 2 Jahre, vier Patienten länger als 3 Jahre und sechs Patienten länger als 4 Jahre nachbeobachtet. Abgesehen von den beiden oben beschriebenen Patienten kam es – beurteilt anhand der Auskultation, des Röntgenbefundes und der Farbstoffverdünnungskurve – in keinem weiteren Fall zu einer Dislokation des Pfropfes oder einer Rekanalisation des Ductus. Das röntgenologisch bestimmte Herzvolumen nahm von 824 ± 238 ml/1,73 m^2 auf 712 ± 187 ml//1,73 m^2 ab (Herzvolumenbestimmungen vor und nach Ductus-Verschluß lagen bei 21 Patienten vor).

Diskussion

Im Kindesalter entwickelt sich bei vielen Patienten mit einem Ductus Botalli eine reaktive pulmonale Hypertonie im Sinne einer Eisenmenger-Reaktion. Diese Kinder erreichen meist nicht das Erwachsenenalter. Ist jedoch der Links-Rechts-Shunt geringer, so kommt es nicht zu einer reaktiven Umwandlung des Lungenstrombettes. Diese Patienten erreichen das Erwachsenenalter, die Diagnose wird dann nicht selten anläßlich einer Routineuntersuchung gestellt. In höherem Lebensalter kann infolge der Volumenbelastung des linken Ventrikels eine Herzinsuffizienz auftreten. Deshalb ist bei einem bedeutsamen Links-Rechts-Shunt aus hämodynamischen Gründen ein Ductus-Verschluß indiziert. Ein kleinerer Ductus sollte wegen des Risikos einer Ductitis oder Endokarditis verschlossen werden [7–9]. Operativ geschieht dies meist durch eine Ligatur. Im Kindesalter handelt es sich um eine technisch einfache und komplikationsarme Operation. Es kommt jedoch, wie auch bei unseren drei voroperierten Patienten, in einer Häufigkeit von 3–10 % zu einer Rekanalisation [7, 8, 18]. Bei älteren Patienten ist die Operation technisch schwierig, weil der Ductus nicht selten stark fibrosiert oder verkalkt ist [12, 18, 30].

Die von Porstmann und Mitarbeitern [20] entwickelte transfemorale Verschlußtechnik hat bisher wenig Verbreitung gefunden. Ihr Nachteil besteht darin, daß ein relativ großer Applikator in die Femoralarterie eingeführt werden muß. Da bei Kindern die Femoralarterie verhältnismäßig englumig ist, ist das Verfahren deshalb erst jenseits des sechsten Lebensjahres anwendbar. Doch auch bei Erwachsenen kann bei einem sehr großen Ductus die dadurch erforderliche Größe des Applikators Probleme bereiten. Nach unseren Erfahrungen hat es sich als vorteilhaft erwiesen, primär eine Arteriotomie vorzunehmen, wenn der Durchmesser des Ductus und damit der Durchmesser des Applikators dem Durchmesser der Femoralarterie nahekommt oder ihn übertrifft. Das Fangen des von der arteriellen Seite her eingeführten Drahtes und das Legen einer arterio-transduktal-venösen Drahtschiene bereitete demgegenüber technisch keine Schwierigkeiten.

Der Ductus sollte konische oder zumindest zylindrische Gestalt haben. Ein sehr kurzer Ductus kann ebensowenig wie ein aortopulmonales Fenster durch einen Ivalon-Pfropf verschlossen werden. Ein derartiger fensterähnlicher Ductus ist jedoch im Erwachsenenalter nach unseren Erfahrungen und denen anderer Autoren [26] sehr selten. Nach tierexperimentellen Befunden [16] kommt es im Laufe einiger Monate zu einer bindegewebigen Infiltration des Ivalon. Der Kunststoff wird allmählich abgebaut und durch Bindegewebe ersetzt, so daß nur das Stahlgerüst im dann bindegewebig verschlossenen Ductus verbleibt. Dadurch ist eine spätere Endokarditis unwahrscheinlich, sie wurde bisher in der Literatur nicht beschrieben. Subfebrile Temperaturen in den Tagen nach dem Eingriff sind nach unseren und den Erfahrungen anderer Untersucher [22] nicht Folge einer bakteriellen Infektion. Vielmehr müssen sie als Reaktion auf das implantierte Material gedeutet werden. Stets kommt es nach einigen Tagen zur Normalisierung der Körpertemperatur. Eine antibiotische Therapie ist nicht erforderlich.

Bei drei unserer Patienten war der Pfropf zu klein bemessen und ließ sich nicht im Ductus verankern. Das ist jedoch unproblematisch, da er zur venösen Seite durchgeschoben und hier in Lokalanästhesie aus der Vena femoralis entfernt werden kann [19–22]. Bei zwei weiteren Patienten dislozierte der Pfropf erst zwei bzw. sieben Wochen später in die Pulmonalarterie. Dies verursachte bei beiden Patienten nur wenig bzw. gar keine Beschwerden. Beim einen wurde der Ductus operativ, beim anderen wiederum durch einen Ivalon-Pfropf verschlossen. Bei der Pfropfdislokation nach Abschluß des Eingriffs handelt es sich um eine ungewöhnliche, in der Literatur bisher nicht beschriebene Komplikation. Zu deren Vermeidung sollte der Durchmesser des Pfropfes 20–30% größer als der Ductus-Durchmesser sein. Seitdem wir so verfahren, ist eine derartige Komplikation nicht mehr aufgetreten. Wenn sich während des Eingriffs herausstellt, daß der Pfropf zu groß ist, muß der Eingriff abgebrochen werden. Der Pfropf embolisiert in eine Beckenarterie und kann hier mit einem Fogarty-Katheter entfernt werden [22, 26, 29].

Unsere Ergebnisse bestätigen die günstigen Erfahrungen anderer Zentren mit dem transfemoralen Ductus-Botalli-Verschluß nach Porstmann. Andere Autoren berichteten über eine Erfolgsrate von 92–95% und eine Komplikationsrate von 5–10% [11, 22, 26]. Dabei handelte es sich meist um leicht beherrschbare Komplikationen noch während des Eingriffes. Todesfälle sind bisher nicht aufgetreten. Alternative nicht-operative Verschlußtechniken wie der Verschluß durch kleine Dacronbespannte Schirmchen [25] oder durch einen Silikon-Ballon [6, 31] befinden sich noch im Stadium der Erprobung und sind durch eine hohe Embolierate von 15–23% [1, 6, 15, 25] belastet.

Literatur

1. Bash SE, Mullins CE: Insertion of patent ductus arteriosus occluder by transvenous approach. A new technique. Circulation 70 Suppl 2 (1984) 285
2. Bussmann W-D, Sievert H, Kaltenbach M: Transfemoraler Verschluß des Ductus arteriosus persistens. Dtsch und Wschr 109 (1984) 1322
3. Campbell M: Natural history of persistent ductus arteriosus. Brit. Heart J 30 (1968) 4
4. Dooley K: Management of the premature infant with a patent ductus arteriosus. Pediat Clin Amer 31 (1984) 6
5. Dudell G, Gersony W: Patent ductus arteriosus in neonates with severe respiratory disease. J Pediat 104 (1984) 915
6. Endrys J, Simo M, Valliattu J, Yousof AM, Khan NA, Zanouna YA: New technic of percutaneous closure of patent ductus arteriosus by a detachable balloon. Circulation 76 Suppl 4 (1987) 45
7. Fisher R, Moodie D, Sterba R, Gill C: Patent ductus arteriosus in adult – long-term folow-up. Nonsurgical versus surgical treatment. J Amer Coll Cardiol 8 (1986) 280
8. Gross R: The patent ductus arteriosus. Amer J Med 42 (1952) 472
9. Gross R, Hubbard J: Surgical ligation of a patent ductus arteriosus. J Amer med Ass 112 (1939) 729
10. Kaltenbach M, Schulz W: Kineangiographische Bestimmung von Ventrikelvolumina mit Rechnerhilfe. Dtsch med Wschr 100 (1975) 590
11. Kitamura S, Sato K, Naito Y, Shimizu Y, Fujino M, Oyama C, Nakano S, Kawashima Y: Plug closure of patent ductus arteriosus by transfemoral catheter method. Chest 70 (1976) 631
12. Kron I, Harman P, Finkelmeier B, Nolan S: The adult ductus. Ann Surg 10 (1983) 546
13. Krovetz LJ, Warden HE: Patent ductus arteriosus. An analysis of 515 surgically proved cases. Dis Chest 42 (1962) 46
14. Latson L, Cheatam J, Kugler J, Gumbiner C, Hofschire P: Catheter closure of patent ductus arteriosus. J Amer Coll Cardiol 9 (1987) 131
15. Lock J, Bass J, Lund G, Rysavy J, Lucas R: Transcatheter closure of patent ductus arteriosus in piglets. Amer J Cardiol 55 (1985) 826
16. Mai J, Hackensellner HA, Porstmann W: Zur Reaktion der Gefäßwand auf die intravasale Applikation von Ivalon. Frankfurt Z Path 77 (1967) 252
17. Merritt A, DiSessa T, Feldmann B, Kirkpatrick S, Gluck L, Friedmann W: Closure of the patent ductus arteriosus with ligation and indomethacin. A consecutive experience. J Pediat 93 (1978) 4
18. O'Donovan T, Beck W: Closure of complicated patent ductus arteriosus. Ann thorac Surg 25 (1978) 463
19. Porstmann W, Wierny L: Percutaneous transfemoral closure of the patent ductus arteriosus – an alternative to surgery. Semin Roentgenol 16 (1981) 95
20. Porstmann W, Wierny L, Warnke H: Der Verschluß des Ductus arteriosus persistens ohne Thorakotomie. Thoraxchirurgie 15 (1967) 199
21. Porstmann W, Wierny L, Warnke H: Der Verschluß des Ductus arteriosus persistens ohne Thorakotomie (2. Mitteilung). Fortschr Röntgenstr 109 (1968) 133
22. Porstmann W, Wierny L, Warnke H, Gerstberger G, Romaniuk A: Catheter closure of patent ductus arteriosus. Radiol Clin N Amer 9 (1971) 203
23. Quian JQ: Closure of persistens ductus arteriosus without thoracotomy. Chung-Hua Hsin Hsueh Kuan Ping Tsah Chin Peking 12 (1984) 101
24. Rashkind WJ: Transcatheter treatment of congenital heart disease. Circulation 67 (1983) 711
25. Rashkind W, Mullins C, Hellenbrand W, Tait M: Nonsurgical closure of patent ductus arteriosus. Clinical application of the Rashkind PDA occluder system. Circulation 75 (1987) 583
26. Sato K, Fuijino M, Kozuka T, Naito Y, Kitamura S, Nakano S, Ohyama C, Kawashima Y: Transfermoral plug closure of patent

ductus arteriosus. Experience in 61 consecutive cases treated without thoracotomy. Circulation 51 (1975) 337

27. Sievert H, Bussmann WD, Kaltenbach M: Closure of left-to-right shunts by catheter techniques. In Hilger HH, Hombach V, Rashkind WJ (Ed): Invasive Cardiovascular Therapy (Martinus Nijhoff: Dordrecht-Boston-Lancester 1987) 25

28. Sievert H, Niemöller E. Bussmann WD, Kober G, Kaltenbach M. Ein Katheter zur Darstellung des Ductus arteriosus persistens. Z Kardiol (im Druck)

29. Takamiya M, Tadokoro M, Okada Y: Nonsurgical closure of PDA. Report of 23 cases J Jap Ass thorac Surg 21 (1973) 196

30. Trippestad A, Efskind L: Patent ductus arteriosus. Scand J thorac cardiovasc Surg 6 (1972) 38

31. Warnecke I, Frank J, Mohle R, Lemm W, Bücherl ES: Transvenous double-balloon occlusion of the persistent ductus arteriosus. An experimental study. Pediat Cardiol 5 (1984) 79

Dr. H. Sievert, cand. med. E. Niemöller, K. P. Köhler, W. Bamberg, cand. med. H. Hanke, Prof. Dr. M. Kaltenbach, Prof. Dr. W.-D. Bussmann, Abteilung für Kardiologie, Zentrum der Inneren Medizin der Universität; Prof. Dr. P. Satter, Abteilung für Herz-, Thorax- und Gefäßchirurgie, Zentrum der Chirurgie der Universität, Theodor-Stern-Kai 7, 6000 Frankfurt/Main 70

Appendix

Selektive Koronarangiographie und Ventrikulographie

Name		Alter	Station

Größe	cm	Gewicht	kg	KO	m²	Datum

Ausgeglichener koronarer Versorgungstyp

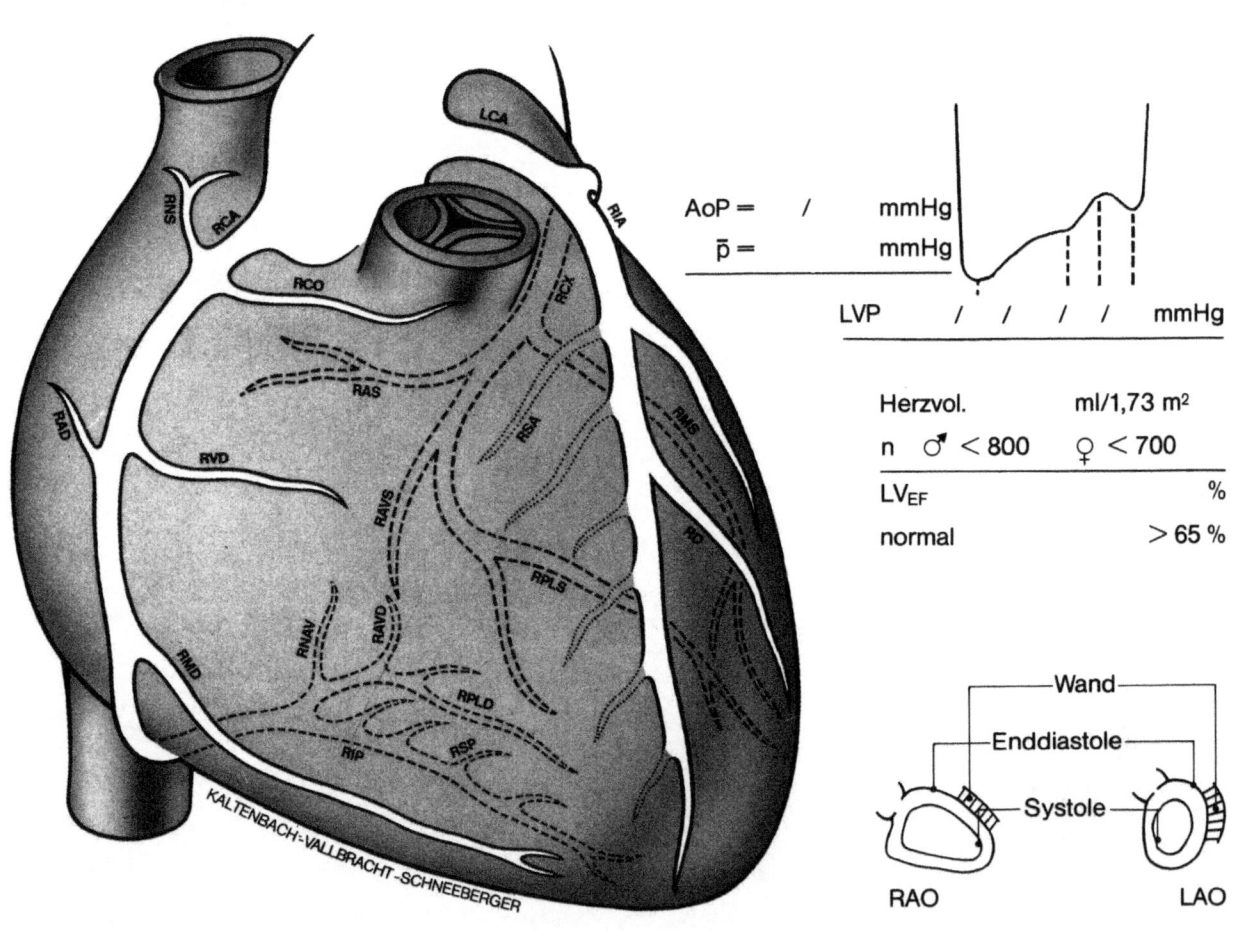

AoP =   /   mmHg

p̄ =   mmHg

LVP   /   /   /   /   mmHg

Herzvol.   ml/1,73 m²

n   ♂ < 800   ♀ < 700

LV$_{EF}$ %

normal   > 65 %

Wand

Enddiastole

Systole

RAO   LAO

KALTENBACH-VALLBRACHT-SCHNEEBERGER

LV in rechts vorderer Schrägprojektion (RAO)   LV in links vorderer Schrägprojektion (LAO)

Abbildung a

Selektive Koronarangiographie und Ventrikulographie

Name		Alter	Station

Größe	cm	Gewicht	kg	KO	m²	Datum

Ausgeglichener Versorgungstyp mit Tendenz zur Rechtsversorgung

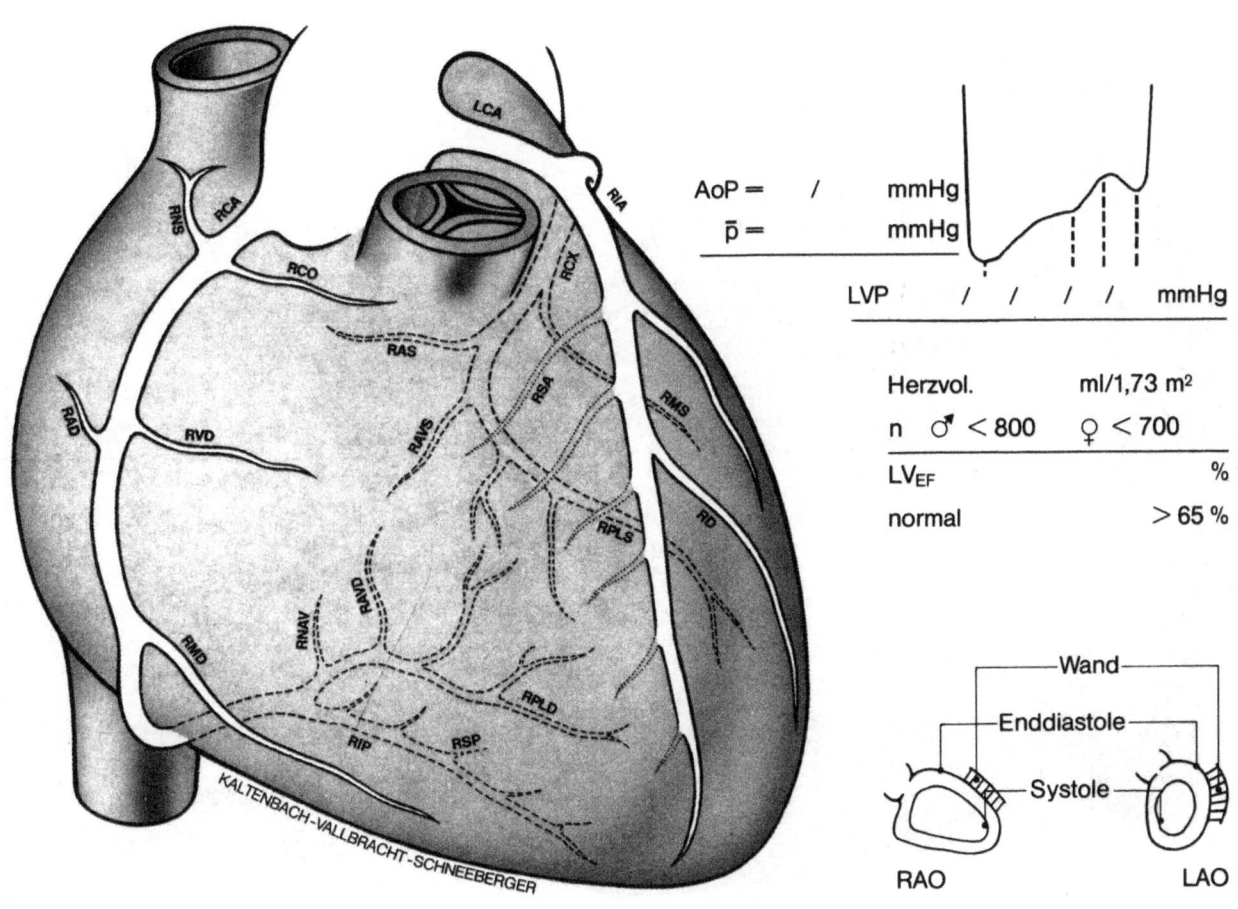

AoP = / mmHg

$\bar{p}$ = mmHg

LVP / / / / mmHg

Herzvol. ml/1,73 m²

n ♂ < 800 ♀ < 700

LV$_{EF}$ %

normal > 65 %

Wand

Enddiastole

Systole

RAO LAO

KALTENBACH-VALLBRACHT-SCHNEEBERGER

LV in rechts vorderer Schrägprojektion (RAO) LV in links vorderer Schrägprojektion (LAO)

Abbildung b

Selektive Koronarangiographie und Ventrikulographie

Name		Alter	Station

Größe	cm	Gewicht	kg	KO	m²	Datum

Koronarer Rechtsversorgungstyp

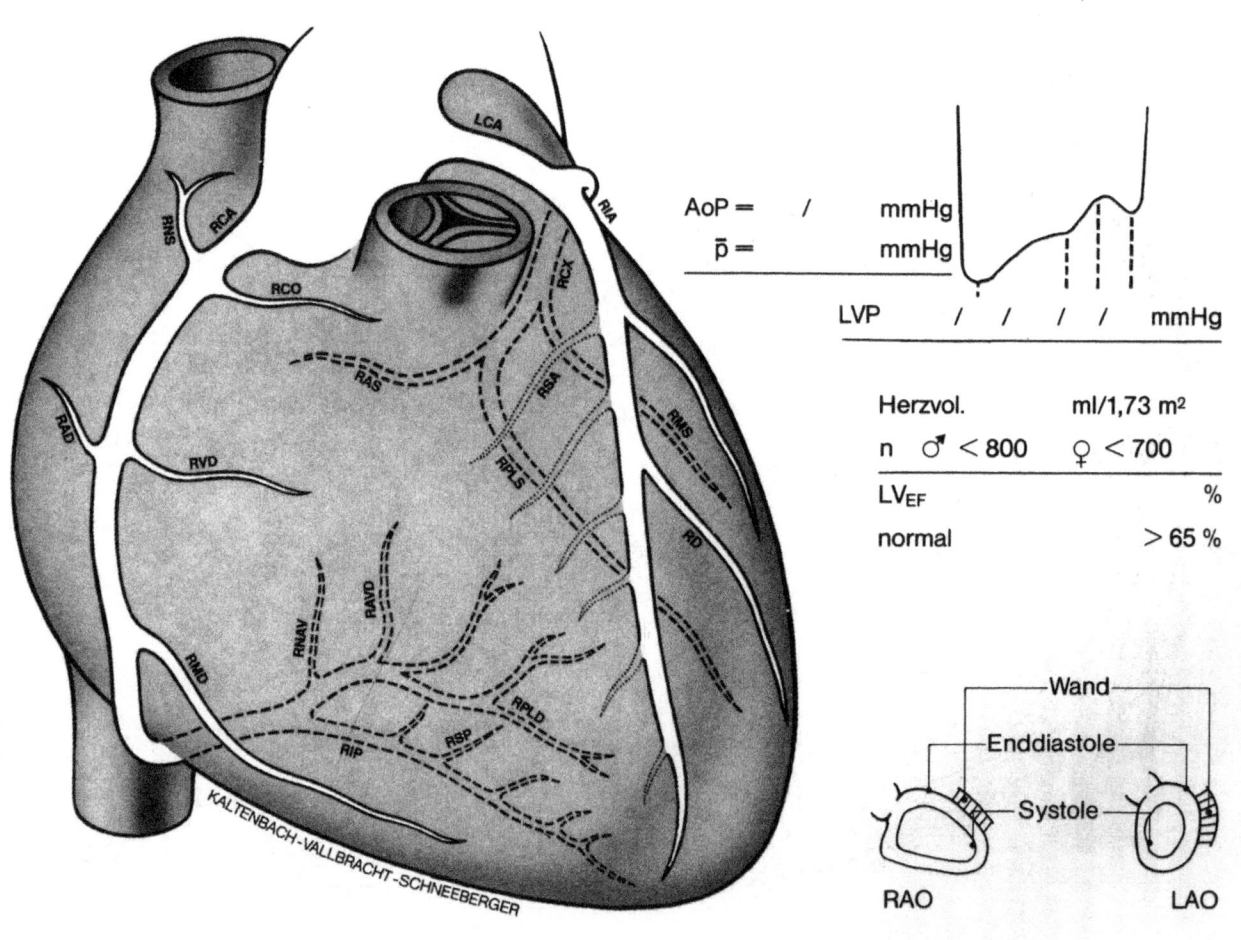

AoP =   /   mmHg

$\bar{p}$ =   mmHg

LVP   /   /   /   /   mmHg

Herzvol.   ml/1,73 m²

n   ♂ < 800   ♀ < 700

LV$_{EF}$ %

normal   > 65 %

Wand — Enddiastole — Systole

RAO   LAO

KALTENBACH-VALLBRACHT-SCHNEEBERGER

LV in rechts vorderer Schrägprojektion (RAO) LV in links vorderer Schrägprojektion (LAO)

Abbildung c

Selektive Koronarangiographie und Ventrikulographie

Name			Alter		Station	
Größe	cm	Gewicht	kg	KO	m²	Datum

Ausgeglichener Versorgungstyp mit Tendenz zur Linksversorgung

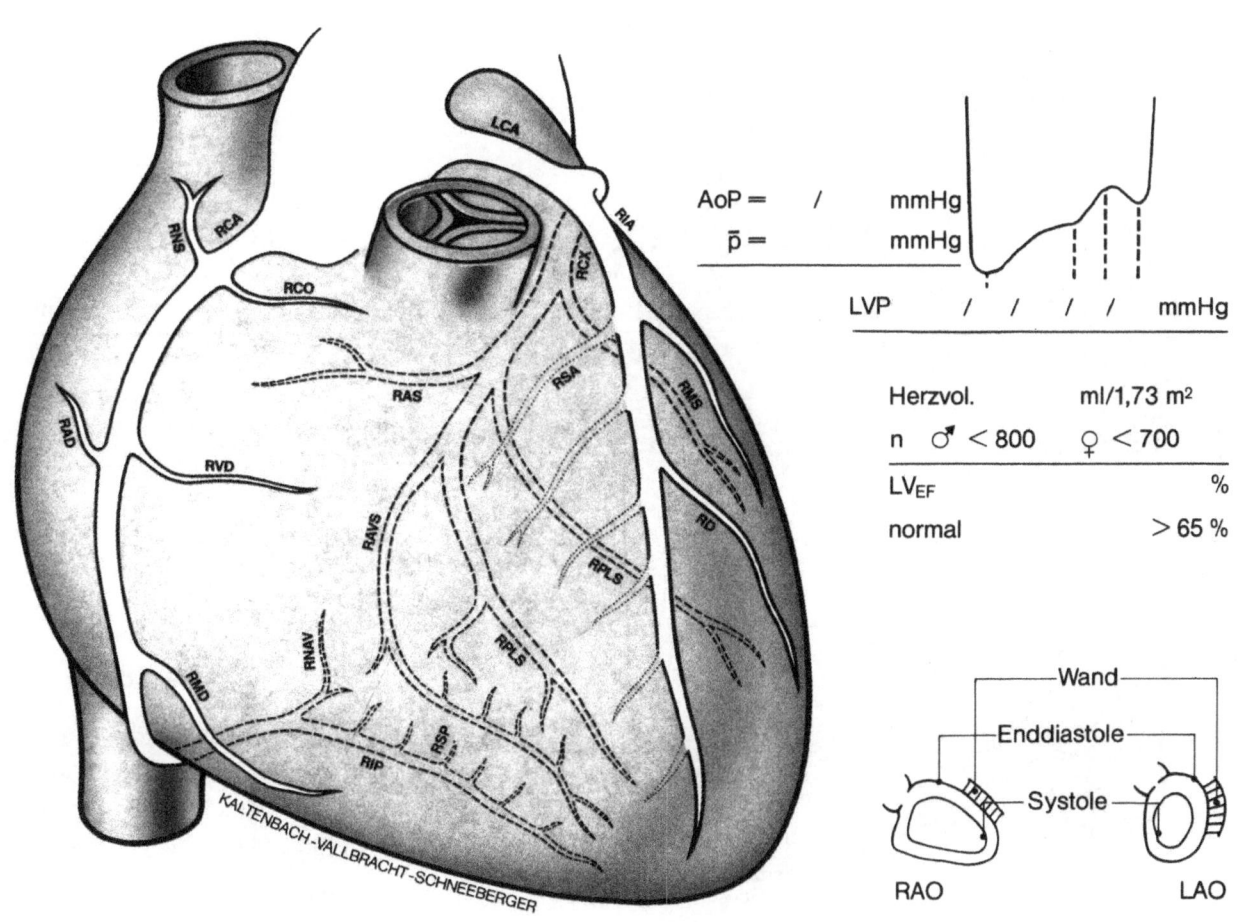

$AoP =$ / mmHg

$\bar{p} =$ mmHg

LVP / / / / mmHg

Herzvol. ml/1,73 m²

n ♂ < 800 ♀ < 700

LV_{EF} %

normal > 65 %

Wand — Enddiastole — Systole

RAO   LAO

KALTENBACH-VALLBRACHT-SCHNEEBERGER

LV in rechts vorderer Schrägprojektion (RAO) LV in links vorderer Schrägprojektion (LAO)

Abbildung d

Selektive Koronarangiographie und Ventrikulographie

Name		Alter	Station

Größe	cm	Gewicht	kg	KO	m²	Datum

Koronarer Linksversorgungstyp

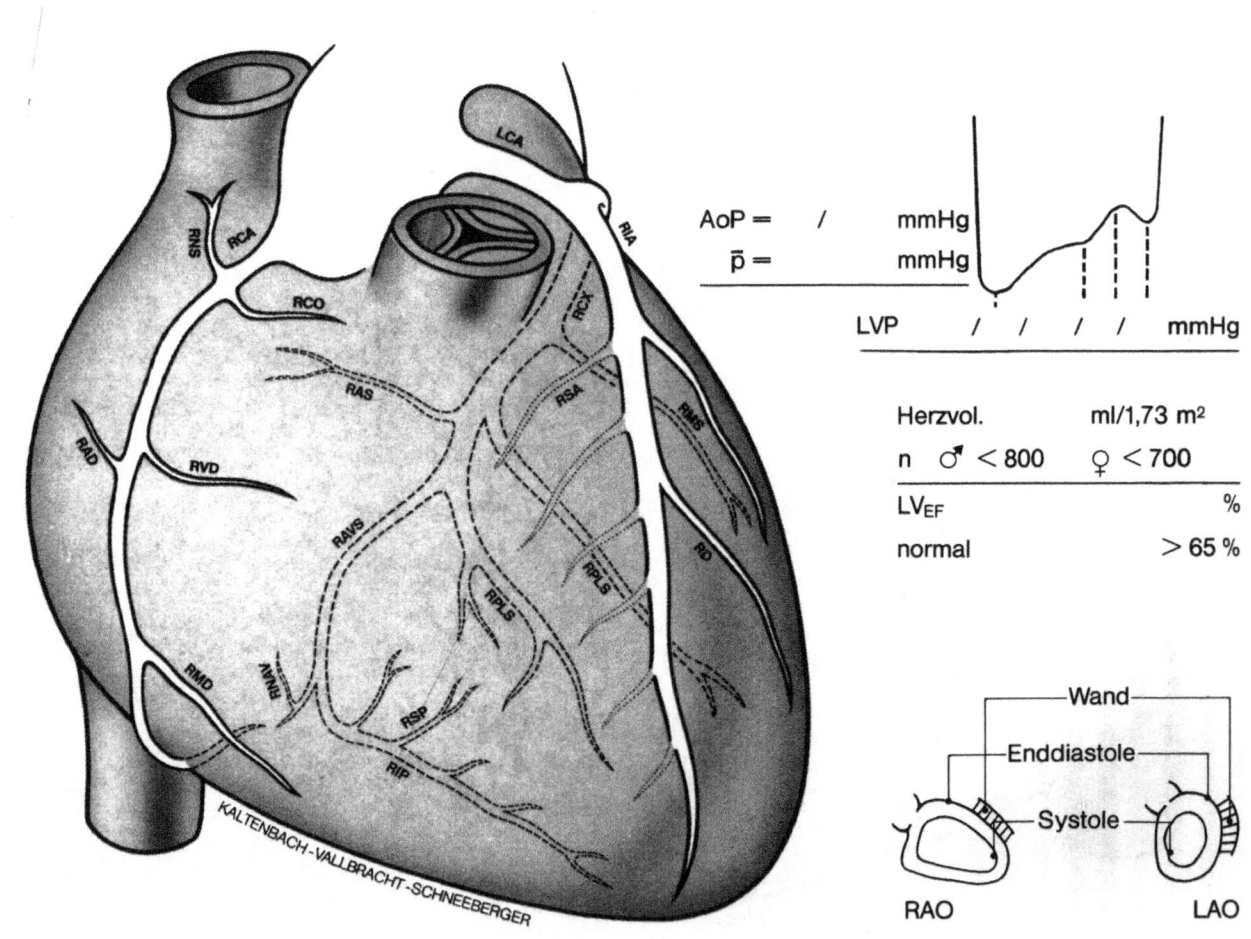

AoP =   /   mmHg

$\bar{p}$ =   mmHg

LVP   /   /   /   /   mmHg

Herzvol.   ml/1,73 m²

n   ♂ < 800   ♀ < 700

LV_{EF} %

normal   > 65 %

Wand — Enddiastole — Systole

RAO   LAO

KALTENBACH-VALLBRACHT-SCHNEEBERGER

LV in rechts vorderer Schrägprojektion (RAO)   LV in links vorderer Schrägprojektion (LAO)

Abbildung e